Looking Good Was Never My Problem

Steps for Living with Metastatic Cancers or Other Chronic Illnesses

Ellen M. Stahl

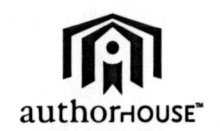

authorHOUSE™

1663 Liberty Drive, Suite 200
Bloomington, Indiana 47403
(800) 839-8640
www.AuthorHouse.com

This book is a work of non-fiction. Unless otherwise noted, the author and the publisher make no explicit guarantees as to the accuracy of the information contained in this book and in some cases, names of people and places have been altered to protect their privacy.

© 2005 Ellen M. Stahl. All rights reserved, including the right of reproduction in whole or in part in any form.

No part of this book may be reproduced, stored in a retrieval system, or transmitted by any means without the written permission of the author.

First published by AuthorHouse 04/04/05

ISBN: 1-4208-3445-2 (sc)

Library of Congress Control Number: 2005903141
Printed in the United States of America
Bloomington, Indiana

This book is printed on acid-free paper.

Note to the Reader: This book is not intended to provide medical or legal advice for people with cancer or chronic illness. It contains the opinions and ideas of its authors. The services of a competent professional should be obtained whenever medical, legal, or other specific advice is needed.

The authors specifically disclaim all responsibility for any liability, loss, or risk, personal or otherwise, which is incurred as a consequence, directly or indirectly, of the use and application of any of the contents of this book.

* * *

Thank you to my dear friend, Donna, who taught me that no matter our health, looking good is not as much about appearances as it is about attitude.

Donna is fighting her own battle
with multiple sclerosis.

* * *

Contents

Prologue ....*ix*

Part I: Own Your Illness *1*

   Chapter One:
   Doing Research 3

   Chapter Two:
   Living in the Medical World 9

   Chapter Three:
   Insurance and Disability 30

   Chapter Four:
   Five Simple Steps to Own your Illness 39

Part II: Heal Yourself *43*

   Chapter One:
   Support Groups 45

   Chapter Two:
   Fatigue and Exercise 49

   Chapter Three:
   Diet and Foods 61

   Chapter Four:
   Spirituality and Meditation 74

   Chapter Five:
   Healing Touch and Other
   Complementary Therapies 82

   Chapter Six:
   Simplicity 85

Chapter Seven:
Purpose and Focus 89

Chapter Eight:
Five Simple Steps to Heal Yourself 93

Part III: Live Your Life 97

Chapter One:
Lifestyle Adjustments 98

Chapter Two:
Love, Sex, and Intimacy 110

Chapter Three:
Attitude Is Everything..114

Chapter Four:
Five Simple Steps to Managing Life with Cancer....122

Epilogue 127

Acknowledgements...129

References and Resources...131

Prologue

*May 26, 1999, late afternoon,
my family doctor's office:*

"The skin of the breast is peau 'd orange – like an orange peel. It is cancer."

May 27, 1999, one o'clock in the morning, alone in the basement, in front of the computer terminal:

"Inflammatory Breast Cancer (IBC): A rare type of breast cancer in which cancer cells block the lymph vessels in the skin of the breast. The breast becomes red, swollen, and warm, and the skin of the breast may appear pitted or have ridges."

Symptoms: "Ridges or pitting of the breast (the skin looks like the skin of an orange).

"This disease accounts for about 1% of invasive breast cancer. The skin of the affected breast is red, feels warm, and may thicken to the consistency of an orange peel. IBC is classified as Stage IIIB … "[1]

No breast cancer is good, but most are more easily diagnosed and treated and have a better chance for long-term survival than does IBC. Mammograms do not detect it. With IBC, there is rarely a detectable lump. It grows in sheets instead of masses. Think of it as your hand with your fingers spread wide apart versus your hand making a fist. By the time IBC is visible in self-exam, the cancer has spread into the lymphatic system of the skin, giving the cancer cells ready access to the woman's entire body. To make matters worse, the inflamed and swollen tissue of IBC is more often mistaken for a simple infection. Misdiagnosis delays treatment for several weeks or months often costing women their lives.

Treatment for IBC begins first with a course of chemotherapy, followed by surgery (mastectomy), radiation, and often more chemotherapy. Because I had fourteen of fourteen lymph nodes test positive for cancer and a bone marrow biopsy also showed cancer cells, I chose to have high dose chemotherapy/stem cell transplant (HDC/SCT) prior to radiation and in place of the second round of chemo. Of all the information I read about HDC/SCT, I've never forgotten this quote: "They [the doctors] take you to the brink of death, then bring you back to life." Well, my life has gone on.

Three years to the day later ...

May 2002, the results of the bone biopsy confirmed metastatic breast cancer was the cause of my severe hip and leg pains. Bone scans confirmed disease in the left shoulder. Low-dose radiation over a ten-day period is scheduled.

More than five years from diagnosis ...

According to Dr. Susan Love, "At this time, nothing we know of can cure metastatic cancer. Thus, the challenge with metastasis is to create the best possible quality of life in the time remaining. We must therefore take a 'management' approach to metastatic breast cancer, which has aspects more closely resembling chronic disease."

Following is my management approach for living with metastatic cancer or chronic illness.

-- Ellen Stahl
2005, Champaign, Illinois

Part I: Own Your Illness

"Warriors take chances. Like everyone else, they fear failing, but they refuse to let fear control them."

Ancient Samurai saying

Owning your illness means you are taking responsibility for it. ~~Whether or not you've been through the various stages of acceptance and denial at an original diagnosis or are going through them for the first time, you should be responsible~~. Your illness and how you choose to live with it is your problem. It doesn't belong to anyone else. You accept responsibility by learning about your illness, building a positive working relationship with your medical team,

Looking Good Was Never My Problem

~~and using your medical and disability insurances to improve your quality of life.~~

Why do you have to own your illness? Don't you have enough to deal with? ~~A~~ *your* ~~chronic illness (i.e. multiple sclerosis) or metastatic cancer~~ does not go away. It does not get cured. Instead, it becomes manageable. The first step to managing this "nasty little business" is to accept ownership of it. *and* ~~Your illness is competing with your healthy cells.~~ Mine is NOT "competing". Mine are already complet[e] mutated and ~~termin~~ from "Agent Orange" 100% complete take over, MUTATED GENES, ~~Whether you use the analogy of a competitive business or an invading army, business gurus or military strategists will advise you to learn as much as you can about the "enemy."~~ and become a warrior. (pg 127)

from birth, through my father, Dan's "direct exposure" (direct quote from his superiors in 'Nam) to Agent Orange. My only sibling, older sister, died at age 33 but was recesitate[d] put into the TOP hospital, put in coma for 2 weeks for having a mutated heart". Luckily ONLY needed a pacemaker but cannot do many things she once did on her farm to doing & being a top YOGA GURU & teacher *[top margin, upside down:] Dan, knowing (a.k.a.) "struggle of ANY KIND, died, in that he word I've been able to possibly help me. Showing absolute zero evidence, and common or so?*

[left margin, sideways:] I AM NOW TOO LATE for ANY form of life. The Government took it upon themselves HAVE EXASPERATED ALL TREATMENTS THAT MAY HAVE HELPED now can only behave sluggish to finding "life, No Fix" is to look and investigate. His demise

[right margin, sideways:] who has the upmost specialized in A.D. doctors in the world. having one of THE ULTIMATE BEST WEEKEND with 2016, Aug 28th, while I, he took a NAP while I went down to do laundry. Within that 1/2 hr or so The V.A. system. Dan, just him and corrections to the V.A.

Dan's every day heartbreak
was knowing that you're,
"he did this to his child."
Later on with Danielle's heart issues
"he did THIS to his children."
(Of course neither my sister and I
had NEVER remotely EVER blaimed
him.)
Then,... it took his own life.

Chapter One:
Doing Research

...Which truly indeed does mean my
horrific, and much worse, case of mutated
A.D. is a done deal. Government not at fault.

When you are diagnosed with a cancer or chronic illness, there are many places to find more information. From the doctors' offices, to the local branch of a national organization, to the library, to a support group at a nearby church, there are dozens of places for you and your family to learn about what is or will be happening to you. It is essential that you not hide your head in the sand or pretend that nothing bad will happen. Debilitating diseases from cancer to multiple sclerosis are difficult to deal with. Prepare yourself for what may come.

who I can ONLY hope my new "serrogate
Dad's", (who call me their daughter, I now
truly call them that.), who were also exposed,
find how to cope with this, not only phyically.
Because I NEED them, especially, as I need as
much help over A.D. that Trump refuses to let ME

[bottom:] of that. Which she adored. You can't get higher than a OUR WEDDG. I've lost much more but this ALL hurts the most

Internet

Today, the Internet is probably the most common source of information. With a little practice and a lot of patience using search engines, it is possible to find information on the disease, the medicines and treatment protocols available, clinical trials, and even to connect with chat groups or on-line support networks with other people facing the same illness. What is especially beneficial using the Internet is the worldwide access. A local support group or even local branch of a national organization does not have the exposure you can get from a worldwide audience. With an unlimited storehouse of information, you can spend significant time in front of your computer.

Since my initial diagnosis, I've used the Internet for medical and drug updates. I've gotten information on what the results of the various blood tests mean. I've used the Internet to find out more about the spine, so that I can understand the difference between lumbar and thoracic regions. I used the Internet to find out about my disability options with Social Security. I also use the Internet to monitor my doctor's recommendations. It is not uncommon for me to bring in pages of information for my semi-annual checkups. I don't have a type of

Part I: Own Your Illness

breast cancer that doctors see on a regular basis. I want to stay as "on top" of the current medical information. Own your illness.

I have used several Internet sites as references throughout this book. These sites were located using one of the common search engines. You will find sites that may or may not agree with the information in this book. Frankly, you may even find Internet information that is not accurate. Apply common sense to what you find; verify information with the appropriate professionals; continue to research. The references cited in this book are not intended to be endorsements or otherwise advocate one web site in preference over another.

Doctor's Office

Oncology (cancer) doctor's offices are filled with pamphlets and handouts from national and local resources. Drug companies often provide information, including relaxation CDs, calendars, and journals. Larger clinics may even have special staff on hand to provide patient education and/or counseling. If you genuinely want to know something, ask about it. The worst that will happen is that you won't get an answer. You will be no worse off than you were before you asked the question. I know there are some people who just want to wear blinders and don't want to know the worst that could happen. I can respect their point of view, but do not advocate it. It is easier to deal with what you know than what you don't know.

National Organizations

There are generic cancer groups, like the American Cancer Society, and specific cancer groups, like the Susan G. Komen Breast Cancer Foundation. Most groups offer on-line and printed materials. Some have local chapters that include support groups. All of them provide opportunities to get involved in fundraising activities. Many groups develop their own "personality." The information is worthwhile and your participation may be just what you need to feel involved with your illness. It is a great way to stay on top of new information that you will need as your disease progresses. Also of importance, you may find a great deal of personal satisfaction devoting your energies to helping others and finding a cure.

Libraries

The first few days after I was diagnosed, I needed to find out just what I was dealing with. So, I went to the library and pulled every book they had about breast cancer off the shelves. Each one had only a paragraph or two on inflammatory breast cancer, so it took several books to get any information. The library had a policy of not re-shelving, so I left the books on the table. That afternoon, my daughter went to the library to help a friend with a term paper. When she came home, she commented about how sad it was that someone must have just found out she had cancer. She and her friend had sat at the same table where I had been. We hadn't told our daughter of my diagnosis because she was just starting her junior year finals and was taking the SAT exam that week.

If you are not Internet savvy, the library is a good place to get help or use a computer if you don't own one.

Support Groups/Organizations

The best information you can get from support groups and organizations is the nitty-gritty things you need to know about dealing with side effects and other problems. Typical research/scientific type books rarely touch on the personal subjects. Do you want to know what a Blood-Richardson grade II; nuclear score 2 and mitotic score 1 means? Check the library books. Do you want to know what cream/gel works best during radiation? Talk to the folks in a support group.

You can also magnify the results of any research you need by working with the members in your support group. There may be people who have already done the research on milk thistle or another alternative therapy. Along those lines, support group members are excellent references for alternative practitioners. While it is just one person's opinion, you can use that information to determine if that option may be right for you.

Chapter Two:
Living in the Medical World

You need to become a team manager when you live with chronic illness. It isn't as glamorous as a major league baseball team manager, and there aren't any exciting perks, but it is a critical role and one you must take seriously.

You need to manage your medical team. You manage the doctors, from your oncologist or neurologist to your family doctor and all the specialists in between. You manage the nurses, the appointment clerks and the insurance clerks. You manage your pharmacists and therapists. You manage your caregivers. You are in charge of them all.

Now, by "in charge," I don't mean you make the hiring and firing decisions (although you do often have

Looking Good Was Never My Problem

a choice of doctors, but the support staff stays with them) or decide how much they get paid. You are in charge of the communication channels between you and your team.

I don't know the statistics, but I suspect it is rare to find a patient with a chronic illness who doesn't have another medical problem like high blood pressure, diabetes, or high cholesterol. Everyone gets a cold or sinus infection now and then. You don't expect your family doctor to treat your cancer and you shouldn't expect your oncologist to treat your high cholesterol. However, the left hand won't know what the right hand is doing without your management. That means you must take a leadership role in communication.

~~Demand~~ Medical Records.

[handwritten: ⭐ One of THE most important things to DO. Part of if you have to.]

Medical records, while they may reside in your clinic or hospital, are yours. It is important that you have these records to manage your illness. Of course, like everything else, managing your records can become a full-time job. Keep in mind just three things, and this job becomes easier: laws and personal preference regarding confidentiality, your right to copies, and your medical notebook. I'll have more to say about your medical notebook later in this chapter.

Part I: Own Your Illness

Confidentiality

Confidentiality applies differently to family and friends and your medical team.

Since my initial diagnosis, we've followed the "no secrets" policy with my family and closest friends. Sometimes I wait until after I have test results before I announce that I had another scan or test, but I don't hold back. This may not work best for you. Over the long term, keeping secrets is just too hard. It can cause resentment and confusion. The people who are closest to you do not have the opportunity to respond when you keep secrets.

Remember too, that when people ask how you're doing, they really don't want to hear all the specific details or get a 20-minute whining session about how bad you have it. Learn which friends and family members really want to know. It is wonderful, actually a necessity, to have a couple of people you can have that 20-minute session with.

Patient Records — GET ALL AND ASAP

DEMAND — There are confidentiality issues within your medical team, not so much because of your team, but because of the various laws put into place to protect your privacy. However, for your own good, you need to name at least

THEY ARE *YOUR* RECORDS. PERIOD.
* YOU ARE the FUCKING PATIENT! *

one other person who can have access to your protected health information (PHI). PHI includes appointment information, test results, diagnosis, or treatment plans. Some offices and clinics require their specific forms with names and relationships to be on file. When billing information for a family is on one account, each member will have access to that information. I have found it beneficial to have an Authorization to Release Patient Information on file for "any requested" date of service and for "all clinic and/or hospital records" for my family. In the event that I can no longer request my own records, they will be able to get copies. As your health deteriorates with chronic illness, it is important to have a trusted back-up person authorized to get you copies and records to keep your notebook complete.

Make sure you can get access to your insurance records too. Because my spouse is the primary holder, I could not even discuss my own billing information until he gave permission for me to be a contact person. The key point is to make sure there is a back-up person, either family member or close friend, who has access to both medical/patient records and insurance/Medicare billing records.

When it comes to getting copies of these records, I have been on the extreme end of both types of offices/

Part I: Own Your Illness

clinics. The first clinic I was involved with gave copies of all lab tests, medicines administered, patient consent forms, patient information sheets for every possible visit. I left the office with a complete record of test results and what happened to me that day.

The second clinic does not provide a single copy of any record unless you specifically request it through the records office and pay the per page fee. After three years, I make a game out of it to see if just once I will get a copy of lab results or patient consent for treatment when I ask for it. I'm still waiting.

I'm convinced it is a policy of the clinic/office administration. The first clinic was very proactive in publishing and communicating a Patient's Bill of Rights. The second clinic has undoubtedly never heard of such a thing. Of course, when there are two extreme situations, there are many more that fall somewhere in between. Remember that the medical records are your records. Even if you have to pay for them, request copies on a regular basis.

Medical Notebook

It is important that you maintain an excellent record system of your appointments, tests, test results, contact names and numbers, appointments, medications, and other information pertinent to your illness. I have never known nor heard of anyone going through a prolonged illness that has not had at least one issue with his or her insurance companies or their medical clinics/hospitals. Keeping good records is imperative for dealing with these issues.

Second, you are not the only one dealing with your issues. You have a caregiver, family member, neighbor, or friend who may be called in on a moment's notice to help. A notebook is a one-stop place for everything you need to know.

Finally, if your illness isn't impacting your memory, your medications or just your age probably will. Over the extended time frame of your illness, you simply cannot remember who treated you for what and when. Many of us in my support group could not even remember our oncologist's name. Chalk it up to "chemo brain," but it is real, and it happens. The notebook gives you the current facts. It is a great historical record, too.

Part I: Own Your Illness

Step-by-step Instructions for Making Your Medical Notebook

You can assemble the medical notebook by purchasing a few supplies from your local office supply store or multi-purpose retailer.

Supply List for Medical Notebook
1 - 1 ½" to 3" three-ring binder
1 pkg. 8-tab notebook dividers
1 to 2 business card pockets
1 - 12 month calendar; one page per month
1 three-hole punch
Small pkg. notebook paper
1 to 2 pens or pencils
1 medium to large canvas tote bag

The 1 ½" notebook is good for about one year's information. If you want to include your insurance explanation of benefits and related paperwork, go with the three-inch notebook. The smaller notebooks are easier to transport, so I've found it easier to keep the medical records separate from the insurance records. Usually, you are taking one or the other. Even if you

carry around both, it is no more than the one large notebook.

The tote bag is needed to carry the notebook, perhaps a water bottle, a reading book, tissues, snack crackers, or whatever you take with you to your doctor appointments. Make sure it is large enough to handle what you like to take but not so big that it feels like you're lugging around a suitcase.

Labeling and Assembling Your Notebook

Make the following label headings for your notebook dividers:
- Contacts
- Appointments
- Medications and Treatments
- Lab and Test Results
- Signed Consents
- Living Will and Medical Power of Attorney
- Notes / Journaling
- Miscellaneous

Contacts: This section contains the business card pockets.

Include business cards for each of your doctors, nurses, clinic billing offices, and pharmacy. If you

Part I: Own Your Illness

cannot get a business card for these people, make one up (use the blank side of one from somebody else if you have to) and include their name, phone number, fax number, mailing address, and email address.

Make photocopies of your health insurance and prescription drug cards. Put them in a pocket.

Finally, include the business cards of your family members and friends whom you may need to contact in an emergency. Again, make one up for them if you have to. If you are making calls from the hospital or clinic, it is difficult to remember all the numbers when you are under stress, perhaps having just gotten bad news about a test or procedure. I found it important to have work numbers available too.

If you keep your contact information electronically, I still recommend using the card system for the contact section. Family members or caretakers may need the contact information and not have access to your electronic device. In an emergency, it will be easier to have the information in the card pockets.

Appointments: This section contains your calendar and appointment record.

Include the calendar pages here. Even if your clinic provides a printout of your next appointment, it comes in handy to jot a reminder on the calendar page. It helps you avoid conflicts because all of your medical appointments are in one place. If you have to travel any distance for appointments, it also helps you to schedule as much into one travel day as you can manage.

My clinic provides printouts that include the date, time, and provider of my appointments. Each entry also includes the location, directions to access that location once you get into the building, and any additional instructions required for the scheduled procedure (e.g. do not eat five hours before this test). Any information you receive related to appointments should be punched and stored in the appointment section of the notebook.

Use this section to prepare for your appointment too. What questions do you have? Have any symptoms gotten worse since your last visit? Have there been improvements? Are there new treatment options or medications that you've heard about and what to discuss? Do you need medication refills, referral updates, etc.? Your doctor will appreciate the fact that you are prepared for your visit. By writing your questions down ahead of time, you will be more likely to remember what you want to discuss.

If you travel to an unfamiliar area, you can also include driving directions.

Part I: Own Your Illness

The Appointment section is a good place to file copies of your specialist referrals if you have an HMO or other insurance plan that requires them. I know my referrals have expiration dates. Make sure you mark your calendar so that you allow plenty of time to have your primary doctor submit a new referral so that your treatments are not delayed or insurance payments denied.

Always put the most current information on the top.

Of course, you may have crossed into the electronic age where you keep your appointment calendar and notes on a palm-held device or even a laptop computer. Just make a notation in the medical notebook with the device and password (if any) so that, in the event of an emergency, your caretaker or family can access the appointments.

☆ VERY IMPORTANT FOR THE Rest of Your Life

Medications and Treatments: This section contains your current medication list and your medication history.

The first page in this section should be your current medication record. The record heading needs to include

- your name,

Looking Good Was Never My Problem

- date it was last updated,
- pharmacy names and phone numbers.

> EASIER AND MORE CLEAR AND MORE efficient AND MORE OFFICIAL/Respected WAY is to Pharmacy to PRINT out "active meds" must ask your Takes 3 mins. of yours!

For each medication, include
- medication name,
- medical condition for which you are taking the drug (e.g. high blood pressure),
- pharmacy where you get the prescription, and
- dosage, including the milligrams (strength of the drug, e.g. 20 mg.), how often you take it (e.g. take 1 per day), and if a generic substitute is acceptable

Medications include prescription drugs, over-the-counter drugs (like aspirin and heartburn medicines), vitamins, and herbal therapies.

At the bottom of the record, list all drugs that you are allergic to and include the reaction/side effects you experienced. Keep the medication record up-to-date. Do not rely on your doctor's medical records to be current, especially since you may be seeing multiple doctors. An example of a medication record is shown below.

File one copy of the research/information pamphlets you get on the medicines. Most pharmacies provide a one to two page summary including potential side

Part I: Own Your Illness

effects when you get the medicine. If you don't get one, you can ask for it. You may never need to refer to this sheet, but in case you do experience a side effect or interaction with a new prescription later on, you will have the info sheet readily available.

Get a record from the clinic or hospital any time you receive a medication or chemotherapy. The record should include the name of the drug, the dosage, and (for chemotherapy) the length of time it is administered. Again, you will more than likely be seeing multiple physicians, nurses, dentists and pharmacists who will need to know all the medicines you've been given in order to avoid prescribing something that could cause a serious reaction. If you do not get a written document that you can punch and store in the notebook, use a sheet of the notebook paper to write down the information.

Use this section to track any side effects, even short-term ones. Report them to your health care provider.

Two other points: always bring a copy of your most up-to-date medication record with you to your doctor visits. It is common to be asked to update your medication list at the beginning of each doctor visit. My list of medications is long, nearly impossible to pronounce and spell correctly, and the dosages are too varied to remember. It is much simpler to just hand over

Looking Good Was Never My Problem

> ☆ Keep me as updated as possible. Pharmacy info list IN WALLET, AT ALL, ALL, ALL TIMES ☆
>
> Since we change meds so many, get new printout really
>
> ☆ See my notes/scratches on Page 20 ☆ (Get is seriously so much better for EVERYONE.)
>
> and THROW OUT (or keep, whatever.) OLD ONES. To much CONFUSION IN this "LIFE" already.

Medication name	Medical Condition	Start Date	End Date	Dosage	Results	Reaction/Side Effects

Part I: Own Your Illness

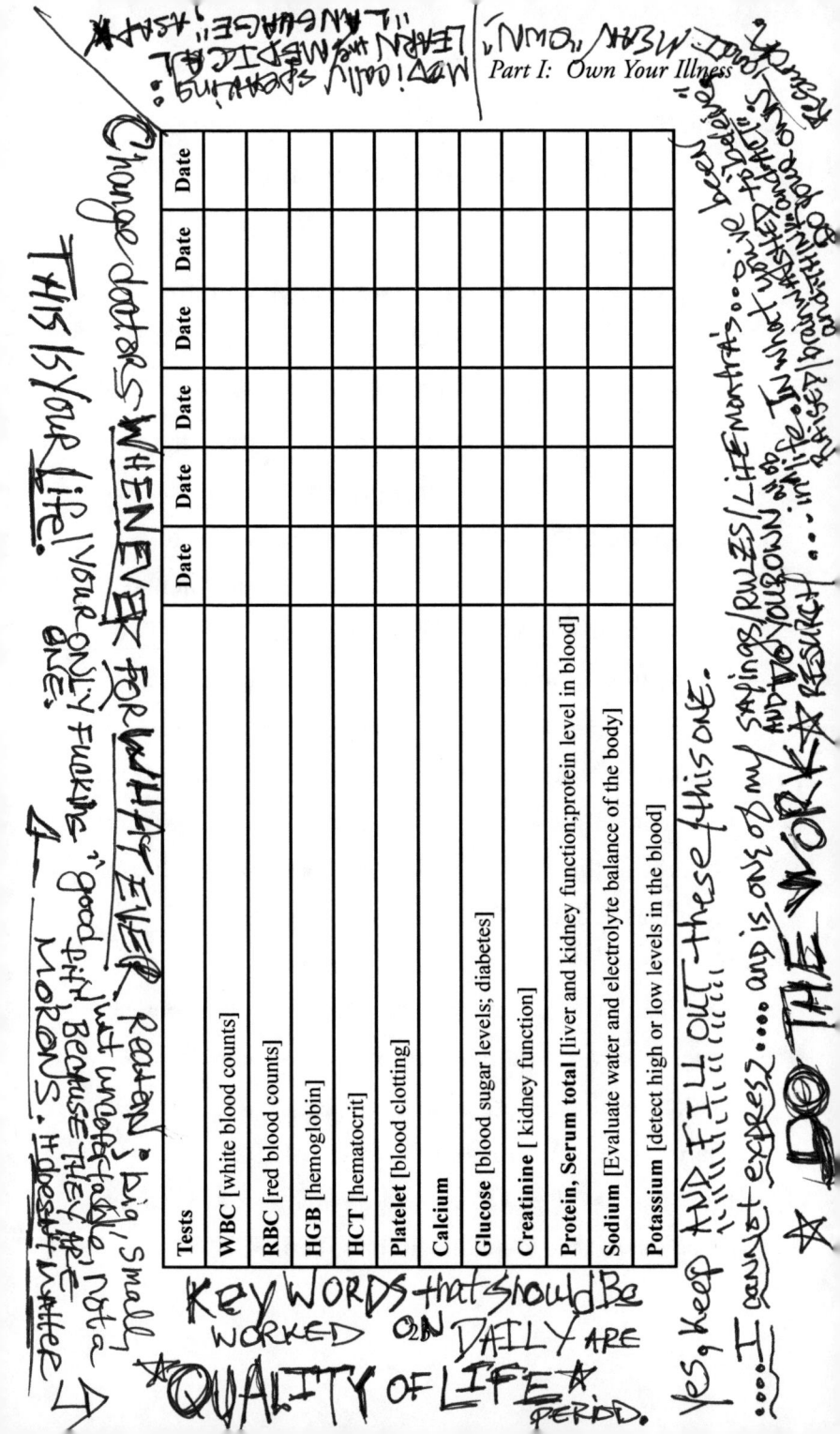

Medically speaking: "MD," "RN," LEARN the MEDICAL LANGUAGE; ASK*

Change doctors WHENEVER, FOR WHATEVER Reason; big, small, just uncomfortable, not a "good fit" BECAUSE THEY ARE MORONS. It doesn't matter.

THIS IS YOUR LIFE! YOUR ONLY FUCKING ONE.

Tests	Date	Date	Date	Date	Date	Date	Date
WBC [white blood counts]							
RBC [red blood counts]							
HGB [hemoglobin]							
HCT [hematocrit]							
Platelet [blood clotting]							
Calcium							
Glucose [blood sugar levels; diabetes]							
Creatinine [kidney function]							
Protein, Serum total [liver and kidney function; protein level in blood]							
Sodium [Evaluate water and electrolyte balance of the body]							
Potassium [detect high or low levels in the blood]							

KEY WORDS that should be WORKED ON DAILY ARE ☆ QUALITY OF LIFE ☆ PERIOD.

Yes, keep AND FILL OUT these / this one. I cannot express.... AND is one of my sayings/rules/LIFE MOTTOS... We began ☆ RESEARCH AND DO YOUR OWN JOB... IN what you have to do ☆ DO THE WORK ☆

Looking Good Was Never My Problem

a piece of paper that can be inserted into your patient file. Second, always take a copy of your most up-to-date medication record with you when you travel.

Lab and Test Results: This section contains the results of lab and other scans, x-rays, and tests.

If you receive regular blood tests to monitor your medical condition, make a chart/table to track the test results on one page. Put this page first in this section and update it regularly. A sample chart for the results of my standard blood work is included. You can make your own chart based on what tests are ordered for you. By including the results for several tests on one page, you are able to see a trend. Many clinics track results this way. Others will just file each test result as it is taken. It is then more difficult to see the trends. While your result may still be within the normal range, has it significantly risen or dropped over the past year? The trend chart allows you to see this information quickly.

File the results of all CT (Computed Tomography Imaging or *cat*) or bone scans, x-rays, or biopsies after the lab results. These results are part of your medical chart. You will probably have to ask for copies of these results. [Refer to the section on Medical Records / Copies on how to get this information.]

Part I: Own Your Illness

Again, if you see a physician to get a second opinion or need the information for another condition, you will have the record available and will not have to wait, often more than two weeks, for your medical file to be copied and forwarded.

Signed Consents: Use this section to file copies of treatment consent documents.

Outpatient procedures, radiation treatments, and even CT scans done with intravenous contrast mediums often require that you sign a "consent to be treated" form. The form provides documentation that the clinic/hospital has, in fact, warned you of any potential side effects of the procedure and you have provided them with any information they need in case of allergies, etc. It provides support for both of you. You should get a copy of any paper that the hospital/clinic wants you to sign. Some facilities are more forthcoming than others. Do not be intimidated by the staff if they make a fuss about getting you a copy. If anything goes wrong, you will need that copy. Trust me, all hospitals and clinics have a photocopy machine. Do not undergo the procedure until you have a copy of the consent form.

If you have any adverse reactions to the tests, such as an allergic reaction to a dye, or a special accommodation is needed, make a note of that in this section too. *SERIOUSLY JUST DO These!*

Living Will and Medical Power of Attorney: Include a copy of both documents.

Many hospitals and clinics like to have a copy of these documents on file, typically if you're being admitted. Your primary care physician may be the holding point for the copies. It is handy to have them in the notebook for the emergency visit or unexpected admission. The hospital can make a copy (at that otherwise hard to find copy machine) or you can give them a copy and make another one for your notebook later.

A brief definition of these two documents is included. The choice to use either of them is up to you. Be aware, also, that the requirements vary by state.

The Living Will *DO THIS ← MAKE ONE! ← NOT HARD*

"Although the term Living Will may indicate that it is a Will, in reality, it is more similar to a Power of Attorney than a Will. Therefore, don't be confused by the title of the document. The purpose of a living will is to allow you to make decisions about life support and direct others to implement your desires in that regard.

Part I: Own Your Illness

Living Wills are needed because advances in medicine allow doctors to prolong and sustain life although the person will not recover from a persistent vegetative state. Some people would not desire to remain in that state while others would. Extending life when death is imminent to some people is only extending the suffering and prolonging of the dying process. The Living Will allows you to make the decision of whether life-prolonging medical or surgical procedures are to be continued, withheld, or withdrawn, as well as when artificial feeding and fluids are to be used or withheld. It allows you to express your wishes prior to being incapacitated. Your physicians or health care providers are directed by the Living Will to follow your instructions. You may revoke the Living Will prior to becoming incapacitated."[2]

The Medical Power of Attorney

"A durable power of attorney for health care [Medical Power of Attorney] is used to appoint an agent to make health care decisions for you and usually includes the power of the agent to make decisions regarding terminal conditions and whether to prolong life. However, if you have a Living Will, the directions of the Living Will control over the durable power of attorney, because you have already made the decision of what is to be done under certain circumstances. Many people use a Durable Power of Attorney for Health Care and a Living Will because they do not want to place the agent in the position of making decisions regarding choice in dying. The agent still has authority to make other health care decisions for you when you cannot make the decision yourself in situations where you need medical attention but are not terminally ill or in a permanent coma."[3]

This book is not advocating or providing legal advice, so be sure to consult with your attorney concerning your needs and requirements for a living will and medical power of attorney for the location where you live.

Notes and Journaling: File some of the blank notebook paper here.

The Notes and Journaling section provides you with paper to jot down information you may transfer to other sections. If an especially caring nurse or technician has treated you, write their name down with a note about what they did so that you can send a personal thank you later.

Part I: Own Your Illness

Often you will have time waiting for your appointment. Use this time for reflection. Write down your thoughts, fears, hopes, and dreams. Sometimes it helps to write these things down in order to face them [fears] or believe that they can happen [hopes and dreams].

This section is also a good place to file inspirational sayings or cards you receive that really lift your spirits or otherwise help you to put your illness into perspective. Jokes, riddles, and pictures that make you laugh all have a place here too.

Miscellaneous: File other information pages in this section.

When I find something new on the Internet or see a new brochure about treatments, I print the information and punch it to fit into my notebook. There may be a clinical trial you're interested in. You can file other information sheets that just don't fit into any of the other sections here too.

If you decided to file your insurance explanation of benefits and other bill receipts with this notebook, the miscellaneous section can be used for that instead. Again, this may depend on the type of insurance.

Chapter Three:
Insurance and Disability

<u>Medical Insurance</u>

Medical insurance is one of the most necessary evils in life. I have yet to experience the joys of Medicare with an insurance supplement, but I am sure they compare "favorably" to the HMO's, networks, and other plans that I have had the pleasure to be associated with.

Actually, I liked the HMO the best. I could manage the regular co-pays per visit and never have to reconcile the bills, especially with my High Dose Chemotherapy/ Stem Cell Transplant with over 30 days in the hospital and a price tag in excess of $250,000. I saw only the $130 charge for television, which I was seldom awake

Part I: Own Your Illness

or cognizant enough to watch anyway. Those were the good old days.

Today I avidly reconcile my EOB - Explanation of Benefits (the statement you get from the insurance company on what was billed to them and how much they intend to pay) and clinic statements. It is a source of great stress. I remember when my father-in-law passed away, I was left with the pleasure of handling his insurance bills. (the benefit of being an accountant!) Of course, in all the mess the one thing I learned is that you don't want to wait too long to file a claim. At that time, we had just six months to send in claims to the insurance company. It didn't matter that the hospital was still billing us eight months later for charges I'd never seen before. I was so frustrated!!!!

When I started with my own lengthy treatments and insurance outside of an HMO, I was determined that every EOB and every statement would reconcile to every appointment / treatment charge. One day a month in this activity and my blood pressure would be up for at least a week. I even tried getting my IV medicine every six weeks instead of the recommended every four weeks in order to eliminate four billing problems a year. Finally, the pain got the better of me, and I went back to every four weeks. Thankfully,

Looking Good Was Never My Problem

at the same time, the clinic fixed one of their billing problems. The "gods" were smiling on me that time!

Insurance reconciliation is compounded when you are covered under Medicare, your primary insurer, and a secondary insurer. All bills go to Medicare first. That is okay, but some clinics will only bill one provider, so your secondary insurer isn't billed. You have to do that yourself. Even worse, there are doctors and clinics that do not accept Medicare assignment, which means you could be in for some very large bills. Take the few minutes to ask your provider what their insurance policies are, specifically ask about Medicare billing and secondary insurers. You may just have to accept their terms or you may be able to choose to get treatment somewhere else. At least you will have the information you need to make your own decision.

From what I've heard from other people, you are either diligent about reconciling your insurance and statements, or you just pay whatever bill you get. Please, for your own sake, be diligent. When you make phone calls, make a note of whom you spoke with, the date, and the time. Most clinics and insurance companies keep note files too, but you need to have your own record. Find out where you can follow-up with a written note. Your written communications

Part I: Own Your Illness

need to include your ID number, the date of service, the billed amount, and an explanation of the error. Be very specific of the action you want taken, e.g. "delete the $200 duplicate charge."

One more lesson I've learned: you seldom get the same answer from the same company concerning the same issue. While I've never had the pleasure of speaking with the same person twice, each person has a different skill set. Don't expect an issue to be resolved the first time, just because the clerk you spoke with said it would be. Follow-up when your check doesn't come in the mail or the correction isn't on the statement. You may find out the first person you spoke with did not research all the facts and the "fix" you were expecting is not going to happen.

It has taken me years to de-stress the insurance process for myself and, truth be told, I'm not 100% successful. Maybe about 50% on a good day. I try not to take it personally. The clinic and insurance company have not singled me out for the sole purpose of making my life even more difficult than it already is. However, I take great joy in the occasional month that the EOBs and clinic bill actually reconcile.

Disability

Sometimes the decision to go on disability is made for you. Your health is just too bad to allow any work activity. Other times, your health is deteriorating and you have to decide if it is the right thing to continue to push yourself to do the same job you were doing before you got sick, move to something less, or take disability.

While undergoing the stem cell transplant, I was in the first group – my health and the treatment did not allow any work activity.

While undergoing both chemotherapy and radiation, I continued to push myself and work as if nothing was wrong taking only an occasional sick day or partial day.

When my husband changed jobs and we moved, I chose to find a job that was less work (both mentally and physically) than I was doing before. It was also significantly less of a paycheck, but it was a choice I thought was the right one.

Again, as my health deteriorated, I continued to downsize my job and paycheck in order to accommodate my fatigue. At least, that is what I thought I was doing. In reality, I was really denying the fact that my illness

Part I: Own Your Illness

had robbed me of the mid-life career that I had always planned on. I was settling for anything instead of facing the facts.

The fact was that I had been on track to achieve the high-level accounting job that I had trained for when I went to college and passed the Certified Public Accounting exam. I was on track to make the move to the level of responsibility that I knew I could handle. I was fortunate that my age was not getting in my way. I was fortunate that the company I worked for the past five years was ready to give me those opportunities. My cancer robbed me of that. It wasn't my fault. It wasn't my company's fault. It was the way it was, but I didn't want to admit it. I wanted to find that mid-life career and was too blind to see that I was taking less and less just to keep working.

So after a year of settling and still being exhausted, I finally started to wake-up. Mind you, it wasn't all at once. More of a slow dawning and some straight talks from a dear friend.

Sure, I feel cheated. But I also know if that is what I focus on I'll be so miserable, I won't even like myself. I did actually even try it for a couple of days. Not too many other people liked me either. That isn't the way to go. I made the decision to apply for the disability and it is the best decision I've made. I have no regrets.

Disability insurance may be available from your employer. If you haven't signed up for it, it may be too late since your medical conditions will more than likely exclude you from it. If you have the option, take it and pay for it.

Social Security Disability is also available. It is not my intent to include all the laws and regulations involved, but it is not a "hand out" program and you should not feel bad about applying for it.

I have disability available from my employer, my employer's disability insurance option, and Social Security. The only place that I did not feel like I was a scumbag trying to take advantage of the system was with Social Security. Perhaps that is because inflammatory breast cancer is a listed illness for Social Security.

The Act and SSA's implementing regulations prescribe rules for deciding if an individual is "disabled." SSA's criteria for deciding if someone is disabled are not necessarily the same as the criteria applied in other Government and private disability programs.

As stated in their website:

Part I: Own Your Illness

"The Social Security Administration (SSA) administers two programs that provide benefits based on disability: the Social Security disability insurance program (title II of the Social Security Act (the Act)) and the supplemental security income (SSI) program (title XVI of the Act).

Title II provides for payment of disability benefits to individuals who are "insured" under the Act by virtue of their contributions to the Social Security trust fund through the Social Security tax on their earnings, as well as to certain disabled dependents of insured individuals."

For other information on Social Security, contact your local office or their website at www.ssa.gov.

When I was first diagnosed and undergoing treatment, I didn't have the resources to understand what I could do with the various disability options from my work or Social Security. It was years later before I knew of Social Security's listed disabilities (applicable to inflammatory breast cancer). I wish someone could have told me – so find a good counselor or human resources professional to assist you. The worst person to talk with is probably your boss (I lost both health

and life insurance coverage doing this). Make sure you discuss all of the following points:
- Short-term disability options
- Part-time work combined with supplemental disability
- Long-term disability options
- Benefits you may lose if you go on disability
- Retirement versus disability
- Social Security disability even if you never worked outside the home

Being on disability has given me back a life. I may not have the high level career that cancer robbed me of, but I have something so much more important. I have the energy to enjoy life without losing the satisfaction of earning an income to help my family.

Chapter Four: Five Simple Steps to Own your Illness

Below are five simple steps to accept your illness with a sense of knowledge, control, and organization.

Step 1: Do your research.

I can spend hours at a time searching websites for information on new treatments, coping techniques, and alternative therapies. But, no matter how much I learn, I will never get a medical degree out of it. What I'm saying is, do your research, learn about your illness and its treatments, but don't get to the point where you are doing your own diagnosis. Have I crossed that line? Well, if I haven't stepped across, I think I've gotten a little too close. Stay on your side, but stay on top of what is happening or can happen to you.

Step 2: Understand your role as part of your medical team.

First, never make the assumption that your doctor, nurse, lab technician, care giver, billing clerk, or appointment clerk know what you are thinking, feeling, or needing. Communication is key to getting the treatments and information that you need. Second, never assume that there is "nothing they can do." Even when you have done your research, there may be alternative therapies or medicines that will help you. After you've mastered the communication part, your only other role on the medical team is to keep the team informed. If you have to do a lot of doctor hopping from one specialist to another, share your notebook – communicate. Oh, and do it with a smile. The people behind the counter may be having a rough day too.

Step 3: Build and use your notebook.

The medical notebook is one of the best tools for understanding what is happening with your illness. It is a valuable tool for you, your family, your caregivers, and your medical team. The medical notebook is a

Part I: Own Your Illness

superstore of information. I have given medical notebooks to friends and family members without cancer, but just to manage their everyday medical records. They all love it, use it, and have thanked me numerous times for it. Take a few minutes now to make a list of the supplies you need.

Step 4: Manage insurances.

Accept that insurance is very necessary regardless of the stress and hassle it may cause. Accept your responsibility in the insurance process. If you have an HMO and need referrals, manage your referrals. Know your co-pays. Use your on-line prescription service. De-stress the insurance process by knowing how your insurance works. Take an active role in reconciling insurance payments with the clinic bills. Mistakes happen, generally not in your favor. Ask for help if you need it. Work with a caregiver or family member once a month to keep your records up-to-date. The worst thing you could do is just drop the statements in the bottom of a drawer and hope for the best. Even I do not have that positive of an outlook toward insurance. If you need to, build an insurance notebook with sections for referrals, EOBs, clinic bills, etc. Organize your papers. You cannot control or change all the insurance rules, but you can manage the process.

Step 5: Decide how disability programs can help you.

Perhaps you are already retired or cannot financially manage on a disability income. Only you can make that assessment. What I can say is that the quality of life I now have is so much better than anything I had either from the money or satisfaction of working. Exhaustion is a horrible way to spend each day. I can now enjoy a few hours, rest when I know my body needs to, and know that I am doing my best. My best isn't what it used to be and it is nowhere close to "doing it all." I don't have to have that anymore. I can do my best and that makes me happy. Happy is a good place to be.

To reinforce what you have just read, repeat the following intentions for managing your chronic illness by owning your illness:

I research my illness and treatments;

I communicate with my medical team;

I manage my medical records and insurances;

I am honest with myself about my limitations.

Part II: Heal Yourself

"Each warrior wants to leave the mark of his will, his signature, on important acts he touches. This is not the voice of ego but of human spirit, rising up and declaring that it has something to contribute to the solution of the hardest problems, no matter how vexing."

Pat Riley

"A warrior without courage is worthless. Do not confuse courage with having no fear. Everyone is afraid; courage is going on anyway. A little fear is good, it keeps you careful, too much fear keeps you from doing what must be done."

Author Unknown

Healing yourself means you are expanding the concept of owning your illness. Healing doesn't mean curing, but it means using your internal resources to better your condition.

Through support groups and simplification, diet and exercise, and finding your focus and purpose, you can heal yourself.

Chapter One:
Support Groups

It is quite simple to find a support group. Most clinics/hospitals offer some type of support group for patients newly diagnosed and undergoing treatment for cancers and other illnesses. The difficulty with support groups comes when you are no longer in one of those two categories. Even though I am not "cancer free" and would be welcome at a cancer support group, I have very little in common with those newly diagnosed and just beginning their treatments. My support needs are different from their needs.

Obviously, I have much to offer the other members of the group, and would never discourage anyone's participation at any stage of their illness, so long as they are comfortable with their role. I participated in a wonderful support group as a newly diagnosed cancer patient while I underwent treatments and found it an enriching and healing experience. My group mirrored the definition and "hallmarks" listed below.

"A support group is usually a small gathering of individuals who share similar struggles. Larger groups may have a common opening session and then break into small groups to allow more intimate fellowship and sharing. Support group members come together at least weekly to share their struggles and their victories as a means of mutual encouragement. The best support groups practice a policy of strict confidentiality so that their members can share freely without fear of others outside of the group learning about their problems.

Here are a few "hallmarks" of a healthy support group:

- Protects the confidentiality of its participants by not disclosing what members share during the meetings to those outside of the group.
- Avoids "cross talk" (interrupting out of turn) and offering unsolicited advice and counseling during the meeting.
- Provides the recovering person with a combination of personal support and group accountability

Part II: Heal Yourself

- Provides a format for honest sharing of personal thoughts and ideas
- Is a safe and non-judgmental environment for the risky experience of exploring and verbalizing emotions
- Supplements the entire recovery process, not the single focus or an end in itself
- Communicates acceptance and freedom of expression without fear of rejection
- Promotes an atmosphere of positive reinforcement and hopefulness
- Maintains a "family" atmosphere into which each individual feels he/she can fit
- Has mature, stable leadership, but is not controlled by one or a few dominant individuals
- Has definite format for its meetings, not rambling, directionless discussions "[4]

I also participated in an on-line support group for inflammatory breast cancer patients, www.ibcsupport.org. Because IBC is such an uncommon form of breast cancer, it was wonderful to email several extraordinary women and their caregivers.

However, as I went through recovery and wanted to get back to what my life was before cancer, I didn't feel good reading the constant stream of emails about IBC. I felt like I was only a cancer survivor or fighter. I didn't want to be just that, so I stopped the support group. I picked it up later, after my first confirmation of metastatic disease, but, again, after a few months, I felt the same way. I know that some women thrive and find their purpose with these groups, but it wasn't for me.

If you are not comfortable with a support group that functions more as a political activist, don't participate. If you find you feel depressed and hopeless after a support group meeting, don't participate. If you find you feel angry, annoyed, or disgusted over one or two members incessant whining, don't participate. Make your own choices about support groups. Make sure you are always 100% comfortable with your group. Support groups are important tools in your recovery; use them wisely to help you. Be careful that they don't drain you instead.

Chapter Two:
Fatigue and Exercise

<u>Fatigue</u>

"Fatigue often is confused with tiredness. Tiredness happens to everyone – it is an expected feeling after certain activities or at the end of the day. Usually you know why you are tired and a good night's sleep solves the problem.

Fatigue is a daily lack of energy, an unusual or excessive whole-body tiredness not relieved by sleep. Fatigue can prevent a person from functioning normally and impacts a person's quality of life.

Cancer-related fatigue is one of the most common side effects of cancer and its treatment. It is not predictable by tumor type, treatment, or stage of illness. Usually, it comes on suddenly, does not result from activity or exertion, and is not relieved by rest or sleep. It often is described as 'paralyzing.' It may continue even after treatment is complete.

The exact cause of cancer-related fatigue is unknown. It may be related to the disease process or its treatments."[5]

Regardless of what causes the fatigue, it is real. It is like running at full-speed and then coming to an abrupt stop. There isn't a slow down period. When you run out of gas, there is no coasting, no cooling-off period. You are done; that's it.

That's not to say you shouldn't stay as physically active as possible. Know your limitations. Use a "day extender" if needed. Don't know what a "day extender" is? It is the "politically correct" term for a wheelchair for those of us who still have mobility but not for an extended period of time.

In all honesty, I have been more in denial of my fatigue than I ever was of my cancer. I can deal with the limitations from the cancer growing in my spine, hips and arms because I can see it on the bone scans and x-rays. At times, I can feel the pain too. I can't see fatigue. Well, I have seen pictures of me taken first thing in the morning and then later in the day. Yeah,

I looked terrible. That is fatigue. Before I went on disability from my job, I would sit in meetings around 3 pm and not be able to follow the conversations. That is fatigue.

I don't know if exercise or the proper diet actually reduces or eliminates fatigue. I do know that both exercise and diet make the time when I am not fatigued better. I feel better and have more energy and enjoying my time is important.

Exercise

Bone jarring aerobics, jogging, and even power walking are not options with my disease. However, moderate walking, especially with our thirteen year-old golden retriever is great. We keep a great pace together (slow), enjoy the fresh air, and don't mind the occasional rest stop. Actually, two little walks are even better than trying to do one long walk.

What makes the walks work, is the fact that I can come home, grab a glass of water, and sit in the recliner for another 30 minutes to recuperate. Every exercise program should include some time in the recliner. ☺

Feel your life force energy

"*Qi* (chi) is the Chinese word for 'life energy.' *Gong* means 'work' or 'benefits acquired through perseverance and practice.' Thus, *qigong* means working with the life energy, learning how to control the flow and distribution of qi to improve the health and harmony of the mind and body."[6]

There is energy in your body that can be moved and focused for healing. The exercises enhance the body's immune system thereby helping the body to heal itself.

Movements require practice but are not difficult. The movements allow the body to stretch and should not hurt. The life energy is opened and moved throughout the body in order to enhance the immune system.

Feeling chi moving through your body takes practice. When you begin to feel this energy, you can direct it with your hands and with your mind to the place(s) in your body that need it the most. Or, you can store it in your **dan tian**---a place about two inches below your navel deep inside your belly—and draw on it when you need to use it.

To get an idea of what chi might feel like, rub your hands together for a minute. Gently separate your hands, palms facing each other, and move them back and forth a few inches very slowly. Feel the push of energy in your hands? This is the type of life force energy that can come into your body through the ground and the air and be directed by the power of your mind to help heal and relax your body.

Life Force Exercises

Both of the following exercises can be done standing up or sitting down. Prepare yourself for doing the exercises with the following "warm-up" routine.

1. Place your feet hip width apart or slightly wider and turn your toes in—you will be slightly pigeon-toed. If standing, relax your knees by bending them slightly. Grasp the floor with your toes and feel the connection of your feet with the ground.

2. Let your legs and ankles become hollow conduits in which the wonderfully grounded and centered energy of the earth moves up into your body.

3. Let your hands rest palms up in your lap or let your arms hang loosely at your sides, your fingers relaxed, and palms facing your body.

4. Put your tongue on the roof of your mouth. This connects the acupuncture meridians on the front of your body with those in the back, creating a full, circular flow of energy through your body.
5. Breathe in through your nose and out through your mouth.
6. Take several deep breaths and feel yourself relax. Then after each inhalation and exhalation, pause slightly. You might want to count your breaths—inhale 1, 2, 3, 4; hold 1, 2; exhale 1, 2, 3, 4; hold 1, 2; etc. Once you establish a rhythm there is no need to count.
7. On the inhale feel the energy come up from your feet through your body. On the exhalation feel the energy run out of your palms or the tips of your fingers back into the earth. There is a lot to remember!

This posture and breath work prepares you for qigong or tai chi exercise. You may feel a tingling sensation in your palms. When you do (or after about 5 minutes of breathing if you're beginning) you're ready to start.

Part II: Heal Yourself

These exercises can be done singly or together at any time of day. For maximum benefit do them in the morning—facing east—and in the evening, facing west.

All movements are gently coordinated with your breath. Breathe naturally and focus only on keeping your mind peaceful and open to receiving healing energy.

Lorie Allen, Healing Touch Practitioner Apprentice, with over eight years of experience with tai chi and qigong, compiled this set of movements.

Exercise One: All Directions

1. Inhale. Raise your hands slowly overhead, your palms facing up, and elbows toward each other.

    Exhale and relax so the elbows point away from the body, palms still up. [If on your feet, stretch up on your toes as you inhale, and relax back on to your feet on the exhale.]

    Breathe in, bringing energy from the air in through your open palms and down through your body.

Stand or sit like this and breathe for a few breaths or a few minutes. Take as much time as you like.

Then, relax your hands in front of you in a "prayer hands" position.

2. On an inhale stretch your arms horizontally out from the body—fingers pointing up, palms pressing out, arms straight. Feel the chi move into your fingers, down your arms and into your body.

    Exhale back to prayer hands.

3. Inhale and push your arms straight in front of you, palms pushing away from the body. The chi moves into your palms and into your body.

    Exhale to prayer hands.

4. Inhale and press your fingers toward the ground at your sides, arms at your sides. The chi flows up your fingers into your body.

    Exhale to prayer hands.

5. Inhale and press your fingers at the ground in front of your toes. The chi moves up and comes into your body.

Exhale to prayer hands.

6. Inhale and cup your hands behind you, arms straight. The chi falls into your cupped hands and into your body.

   Exhale to prayer hands.

7. Breathe in and out several times. On an exhale, lower your hands to your dan tian and store the chi you have just acquired.

   Relax and go on with your day or on to the next exercise.

Exercise Two: Circulating Chi

Many tai chi exercises focus on moving or holding a ball. That thought shows you where your hands should be in relation to each other—just like holding a ball. The size of the ball you choose to hold in this exercise is up to you. I started practicing with an imaginary ball the size of a deflated soccer ball. I like one more the size of a basketball now.

This exercise can be practiced for as long or as short a time as you'd like. When you can feel the energy in just a few minutes, concentrate on sending that lovely circulating energy where your body needs it most. You may not know where that is even if you think

Looking Good Was Never My Problem

you do, so set your intention for the chi to go where it is needed most in your body. When I first started feeling energy, I heard a loud humming—I thought the washing machine was out of balance---and then I felt a wonderful warm, circulating energy in my chest. When I asked my teacher about it he said if I practiced enough I could dematerialize. Then he smiled. I could tell that what was happening was good, but try as I might I still haven't dematerialized.

1. Rest your hands on your dan tian. Bring your palms sky-up and slowly raise your hands chest high while inhaling.

2. Exhale and press your palms away from your body, arms straight. WOW! You found a ball out there! Hold onto it, palms facing each other and on the next inhale bring your hands back toward your chest.

3. Exhale and, still holding the ball, again extend your arms from your chest.

4. Inhale, and bring the ball back toward you, placing your hands on the top and bottom of the ball rather than the sides.

5. Relax your shoulders. Place your tongue in the roof of your mouth. Relax your knees.

Part II: Heal Yourself

And-breathing normally, rotate the ball in your hands as slowly as you can. One hand will move in a clockwise pattern, and the other, counter-clockwise. If you get tired, just slowly change the position of your hands and continue.

Both hands move slowly and the chi builds between them. Focus your breath on the ball. Make it real. Feel the energy building up between your hands—the energy of the ball.

Over time this energy can be directed from the hands up your arms and into any part of your body. You might feel a vibration in your chest and hear humming or other sounds. This is the chi circulating in your body and going to the parts of your body that need it the most.

You can practice these exercises any time you need healing energy, want to meditate, or just need to relax quickly

Remember, the energy is always coming up through the soles of your feet and down from the crown of your head.

Looking Good Was Never My Problem

When you have finished this exercise, slowly concentrate on pushing all the energy into your dan tian.

If you get dizzy or feel there is too much energy, push it quickly away from your body and shake your hands. Start over when you are ready. Storing the energy in your dan tian allows your body to draw on it any time extra chi is needed any place in your body.

Chapter Three: Diet and Foods

It seems that a day doesn't go by when another food is added to the list of cancer preventatives or, conversely, removed from the list. Of course, the good list may also depend on which celebrity or which health guru is the "man/woman of the hour."

Then, of course, is the age-old argument of fresh versus canned versus frozen. Thankfully for all of us, I am not going to add to that debate now. However, it isn't hard to agree that even canned green beans have it over a bag of greasy, fried and salted, potato chips -- at least from a healthy eating perspective if not a comfort food one.

At the basic level, food is energy. Energy is fuel. Fuel fights fatigue. Fatigue plagues chronic illness patients (as well as many others). Learn to use foods to your benefit. My five-step approach to an eating plan follows.

Don't berate yourself over past eating sins.

I knew a woman in her early thirties who was diagnosed with breast cancer. She was the poster child for healthy eating and exercise. She came from a family of less than perfect eaters, all with health problems. Early on, she was convinced if she ate properly (fruits, vegetables, no red meats, no "junk" foods, etc.) and exercised faithfully, she would remain free of health problems. Three weeks into treatment for breast cancer, she had her first slice of pepperoni pizza.

On the other side, I am a perfect example of the bad eater. Not that I have an aversion to healthy foods, but I developed a much closer relationship to comfort foods, like chocolate cupcakes with fluffy white filling and little white frosting squiggles on the top. I'd also been eating pepperoni pizza since I started working in a pizza place when I was 16. Knowing all this, I carried around some guilt that my eating habits might be a contributor to my illness. They still might be. However, the first support group I went to had eight women, all breast cancer patients. Two of the women were "sticks;" two were "jocks;" three were just average; and I was "plump." As I looked around the room, I finally realized, what you eat is not the only factor that contributes to what illness you get.

You can change your eating habits or you can continue doing whatever you were doing before. The key lesson is to know that whatever you eat it is fuel for your life.

Find an eating plan that works for you and stick with it!

My favorite is the "eat all day" plan. Actually, it isn't all day, but it is five to six times a day. Here's the reason. Small meals/snacks go down easier.

Again, I go back to the fatigue factor. When I'm tired, I can't eat. As a matter of fact, I've lost a few suppers when I've been going all day, then finally sit down to a meal, and am just too exhausted to digest it. Second, small meals/snacks keep your metabolism working, providing fuel to your body.

It isn't uncommon to find a diet guru or eating program that follows this concept. My approach isn't unique. This isn't an approach to weight loss, although it could be used as one. This is a practical approach, again to deal with fatigue.

Fatigue Fighter Eating Plan

Breakfast bread/grain/potato fruit	**Morning Snack** fruit meat/fish/dairy
Lunch bread/grain/potato meat/fish/dairy vegetables	**Afternoon Snack** meat/fish/dairy fruit
Dinner bread/grain/potato meat/fish/dairy vegetables	**Evening Snack** fruit

Determine what you will eat.

The easiest diet is one where you just apply commonsense. Too much of a good thing is still too much. Moderation is key. Check packages for recommended serving sizes. If you need to lose weight, reduce your portions. Use salad/dessert plates instead of large dinner plates. Measure cereal, rice, and pasta where it is very easy to exceed serving sizes. A good rule of thumb is that a serving is about ½ cup for fruits and bread/grain/potatoes, 1 – 2 cups for vegetables, and 2 – 4 ounces for protein (or a serving about the size of your fist).

Let's face it. Some foods are just better for you than others. While a calorie is a calorie, good calories will help you feel better and provide the quality fuel you need. Good food choices are in the following table:

Food Group	**Specific Foods**
Proteins	Low-fat or fat-free (only) milks, cottage cheeses, and yogurts Lean meats, like pork tenderloin or chops, beef, white-meat turkey and chicken Fish, like shrimp, tuna, halibut, mahi mahi, cod, orange roughy Eggs
Bread/grain/potato	Vegetables, like jicama, parsnips/turnips, potato (white and sweet), squash, corn, beans (black, red, kidney, lentil, navy) Grains, like barley, oatmeal, rice, rice noodles, pasta Breads and cereals, like bagels, waffles/pancakes, tortillas, stuffing, granola and bran cereal

Looking Good Was Never My Problem

Food Group	Specific Foods
Fruits	Grapefruits, berries, peaches, pineapple, bananas, apples, cantaloupe, honeydew, papaya, pears, plums, grapes, mango, oranges, nectarines, tangerines, watermelon, cherries
Vegetables	Artichokes, asparagus, beets, bell peppers, bok choi, broccoli, brussel sprouts, cabbage, carrots, cauliflower, celery, cucumbers, eggplant, green beans, greens/lettuce, mushrooms, snow peas, spinach, sprouts, zucchini, tomatoes

Out of all of these choices, how do you know what to eat? First, cross off all those vegetables that just don't cut the mustard, even if you drenched them in Grey Poupon. For me that's artichokes, brussel spouts, eggplant, and mushrooms. Do the same with proteins, bread/grain/potatoes, and fruits. Let's be honest, if you don't like it, you won't stick with the plan anyway. Okay, and give yourself a little pity – if things aren't looking so good for your longevity, don't spend that time choking down slimy, gray mushrooms.

Which brings me to another point, is chocolate actually a vegetable? You've seen the "logic":

Part II: Heal Yourself

chocolate comes from the cocoa bean; beans are vegetables; therefore, chocolate must be a vegetable. That logic is right up there with my mother's thoughts on oatmeal cookies. Oatmeal is good for you; oatmeal cookies have eggs in them; eggs are protein; protein is good for you; therefore, oatmeal cookies are good for you. Put chocolate chips in them, and you've added a vegetable! Dip the oatmeal cookies in fat-free milk and they're even better! Enough!

There are actually some foods that are better for you. Foods that add cholesterol (like egg yolks) or sodium (lots of the canned vegetables) should be limited. Canned fruits packed with added sugar are not the best choices either. [Here's a tip on canned peaches: buy *"freestone"* peaches instead of yellow cling. They taste so much fresher and so much less like plastic.] Avoid fried foods. Choose breads made from whole grains.

I like to apply the food information in <u>Traditional Chinese Medicine, A Natural Guide to Weight Loss That Lasts</u> by Nan Lu. He recommends certain foods that heal. For me this translates into using my calories in the best possible way. There is a great deal that goes into the Traditional Chinese Medicine approach, but choosing these particular foods may also be of benefit to you.

Fruits: Kiwis, oranges and tangerines, pears, red apples, red grapefruit, red grapes, strawberries, watermelon

Vegetables: Broccoli, carrots, cauliflower, celery, plum tomatoes, yellow squash and zucchini

Purchase your vegetables off a grocery's salad bar if you don't use up the full-size items. Salad bar prices may be higher, but if you end up throwing vegetables away, the salad bar may turn out to be a better option. Plus, if you just want a little of something, the salad bar allows you to get even a couple of tablespoons to jazz up a recipe.

One final thought on foods. Warm foods are easier on your system. Too hot and you burn your mouth. Too cold and you throw your 98 degree body into shock. I like my salads without the chill. Except for popsicles and ice cream (which isn't on the preferred food list anyway), foods don't have to be frozen when eaten. As my Uncle Mike says, "If fruit was meant to be eaten cold, it would grow in Alaska."

Part II: Heal Yourself

Determine what you will drink.

Have you ever read anything about what to drink that didn't tell you to drink at least eight glasses of water? Well, I don't want to be the first. Keeping your body clean on the inside is just as important as keeping it clean on the outside.

However, a recent article in our local newspaper claims that eight-glasses-a-day advice turns out to be a myth. "In 10 months of searching medical literature and talking to specialists in fluids and thirst, Dr. Heinz Valtin [kidney specialist and retired professor at Dartmouth Medical School in Hanover, New Hampshire] came up dry. He found no scientific basis for drinking eight glasses of water a day or where the idea originated. However, his conclusion applies to healthy adults."[7] So, back to my original statement, drink that water!

Soda pop, even diet and caffeine-free, is not a replacement for water. Green tea, especially with lemon ginseng, is a better choice. Herbal teas, like ginger and chamomile, are great too.

I apply the same thought to cold drinks as I do cold food. Leave out most of the ice. Just a suggestion…

Decide if you will add nutritional supplements.

Even with the best of food choices, when your system is weak or your immune defenses at less than optimum, you may benefit from nutritional supplements, i.e. vitamins and minerals. Consult with your health care provider or a nutritionist to find the right doses for you.

I supplement a multi-vitamin with extra B complex, calcium, Vitamin A, and Vitamin E. B vitamins (Thiamin, Riboflavin, B6 and B12) all help with your metabolism, weakness, and fatigue. Vitamin E is an antioxidant and helps the blood cells. Vitamin A also helps with immunity and bone strength. Calcium is also for bone strength.

There are general guidelines to the benefit of nutritional supplements available on line at www.nutritional-supplement-info.com or in the PDR for Nutritional Supplements by Sheldon Saul Hendler and David Rorvik. Remember to consult with your doctor about adding nutritional supplements to your diet.

Live with your food plan choices.

When I say live, I mean live! Just do it moderately. We have a lovely restaurant in town that serves sweet potato chips and fabulous single dip chocolate sundaes. When we go, which isn't all that often, my husband and I share sweet potato chips, and we both indulge in a sundae.

For your birthday, have a piece of cake. Birthdays and cake are two of the most wonderful things in this world.

Raspberries and peaches are some of my favorites. When they are in season and affordable, I really indulge myself. Enjoy foods in their season. It is totally fabulous and makes eating them so much more special.

If you don't already like to cook, try it by starting with simple dishes. I'm not the world's best gourmet cook, but I do take pride in knowing I've put together a healthy and tasty meal that my husband and I enjoy. A sample of my favorite tasty and simple meal ideas follows.

Quick and Easy Mornings and Snacks

Top a low fat frozen waffle with a combination of fresh strawberries and vanilla yogurt.

A great mid-morning/afternoon snack is a couple of slices of deli turkey and ½ cup of freestone peaches.

Spread a thin layer of peanut butter on a couple of rice or popcorn cakes. Top with banana slices.

Mini-Meals Made Easy

Mix ½ cup canned chicken with mandarin orange slices, green onions and almonds. Use some vanilla yogurt in place of mayonnaise. Pile on a slice of toasted low fat wheat bread. Serve with red grapes.

Combine 1 small cooked, diced chicken breast with 2 cups mixed greens, chopped green onion, ½ cup mandarin oranges, and 2 tablespoons sliced almonds. Mix the orange syrup/juice with vanilla yogurt to get the consistency of salad dressing. Pour over the salad, toss, and enjoy!

Pour 1 can tomato soup over 4 cooked hamburger patties in a medium frying pan (be sure to drain all grease from the patties). Add ¼ cup chopped onion and 1 cup chopped green pepper. Simmer for 15 –20 minutes on low heat. Serve over white rice with a side of glazed baby carrots.

Marinate 24-32 peeled, raw shrimp (remove tails) in a mixture of ½ cup olive oil, ¼ cup lemon juice, 1 teas. oregano, 1 teas. Dijon mustard, ½ teas. rosemary, ¼ teas. crushed red pepper flakes, dash of salt and pepper for at least one hour. Grill for 3-4 minutes (or until

Part II: Heal Yourself

shrimp is cooked through) on a double-sided electric kitchen grill. Toss shrimp in a Caesar salad (use a pre-packaged salad mix to keep it really simple).

Chapter Four:
Spirituality and Meditation

"...the spirit reveals itself to everyone with the same intensity and consistency, but only warriors are consistently attuned to such revelations." Readers and warriors alike, proceed in the spirit of free will to access the power of intention.[8]

Spirit connects you to the universal energy that enriches your life beyond anything you can imagine. Connection with the spirit brings you love, kindness, support, and knowledge at the best times and in the right quantities to benefit you best. Spirit explains why my daughter found the research books at the library,

Part II: Heal Yourself

and why I was connected with a particular customer service representative over 2,000 miles away.

I was calling the customer service group for one of the major hotel chains. We had a reward certificate we would not be able to use because I had to have a round of radiation treatments that caused us to cancel a vacation. I explained all this to the young woman who took my call. Turns out, she was a five year cancer survivor. She had been given little chance of survival but was at work now and in good health. She recommended that I read a book by Dr. Bernie Segal called <u>Love, Medicine and Miracles</u>. I picked up the book from a local bookstore on the way home from my first day of radiation. It was exactly what I needed at exactly the time I needed.

After reading it, I gave it to my father to read. Shortly after he finished it, he was walking his dog and ran into a neighbor whom he hadn't seen for several weeks. Turns out this man was recently diagnosed with cancer and had been undergoing treatment. <u>Love, Medicine and Miracles</u> was shared with another person at the exact time that they, too, needed it. If that isn't a universal spirit at work, I don't know what is.

Spirituality is being able to recognize a coincidence for more than what it seems on the surface. I experienced

Looking Good Was Never My Problem

an interesting encounter several months before my first diagnosis, but definitely when my body knew that it had cancer.

I met him at the Chevy garage. I'd brought our Blazer in for a routine oil change. He'd brought his vehicle in for some routine maintenance too. We sat in the customer lounge, waiting for the courtesy van to take us to work.

I glanced across the room noticing his impatience as he rifled through his briefcase for a specific paper. He found it and headed for the phone.

It wasn't until he finished the sales call that he looked around the room and noticed I was there.

"Waiting for the van?"

"Yes."

"Usually they're right here. I've never waited this long."

"Yeah, I hate waiting but I hate asking my friends or co-workers to go out of their way to pick me up here."

He sat down and closed his briefcase before he replied,

"Sometimes you have to ask for help. You need to learn that. I still have a hard time with it, but you'll have to learn."

"Yeah," I smiled and shrugged, knowing he was probably right but not knowing what else to say.

"Well, my car wasn't supposed to take too long anyway." He picked up his briefcase and walked to the service counter.

A van pulled up outside and the driver popped his head in the door. "Ready to go?"

I turned to tell the salesman that our ride was here, but he was gone.

Obviously, spirit was sending me a message. Look for messages in what you may have considered to be just ordinary coincidences. Soon you will find that you are receiving messages that will bring you what you need when you need it.

Messages can also come from inside you. Meditations can guide the energy inside of you to the part of your body that needs healing. According to authors Deepak Chopra, M.D. and David Simon, M.D, "People who regularly meditate show improvements in their immune function and reduced susceptibility to

Looking Good Was Never My Problem

infections."[9] We need our immune system to fight our illnesses.

A simple meditation requires only that you sit comfortably (again, I go for that old recliner), close your eyes, and slowly inhale and exhale through your nose. I like to think or softly say "light" on the inhale and "love" on the exhale. I am bringing a healing light into my body and sending out love. Chopra and Simon use the words "so" and "hum." If you have a simple mantra that has meaning for you, use it. If your attention drifts or you are distracted by other sounds, continue to say your mantra on the inhale and exhale. It will keep you focused on the meditation and your breathing. Do this for about twenty minutes, preferably in the morning and early evening.

Another type of meditation is guided imagery. Bernie Siegel, MD has a nice tape/CD where he guides you to a special place where you can find whatever it is that you need for healing. These meditations usually take about thirty to sixty minutes. They can be very beneficial when you have a particular spot where your body needs to direct its healing power.

Lorie Allen provides the following ten to fifteen minute guided meditation. You may record it for your use or just read it with quiet pauses for reflection and healing.

Meditation for deep relaxation and healing

Sit or lie down. Be comfortable. Be sure your legs and hands are not crossed and your feet are about hip width apart. If seated, plant your feet firmly on the floor and let your head float calmly on the top of your neck.

Close your eyes and let your palms rest palms up at your sides or on your lap.

Take a couple of slow, deep breaths and feel yourself sink even more comfortably into the chair, floor, or whatever surface supports you. Breathe normally, but slowly and with awareness.

Be aware of the gentle flow of air around your nostrils. The air coming deep into your body, circulating from your lungs throughout your body and rising up from your lungs to leave through your nostrils, leaving your body deeply refreshed. Notice how the air feels at your nostrils. It seems to be made of a wonderful white light. With each breath, inhale the beautiful white light and see it washing through all the cells of your body. Exhale all soreness, tiredness, pain, or tension---all your worries leaving in the clean white healing light. Breathe in the light and exhale your tensions. The light circulates through all the cells of your body, making you glow. Breathe in this way for as long as you like, glowing more and more strongly and becoming more deeply relaxed and calm.

When your body is so full of white light you think you can't hold any more, you notice how deeply relaxed and at peace you are. And you notice that while your body has been enjoying the beautiful light circulating through your entire system, your palms have each collected a large ball of light. Each palm now holds a golden ball of beautiful energy. Energy that lives in the palm of your hand you can now use to help your body become even more relaxed and help it heal.

Take one of your hands now, and place it gently over a part of your body that you feel needs it the most. It may be a place where you know cancer is growing or where cancer once grew. But only love can grow in the beautiful light. And as you place your hand on this spot, spreading your fingers wide, feel the warmth of all the love that the world truly has for you pour into your body. All the cells in your body that aren't made of the love of the white light leave through your outspread fingers. Your entire body, inside and out, glows with the white healing light of love.

Part II: Heal Yourself

Your other hand still glows with the ball of energy it holds. Take this lovely ball of energy and pour the energy into your lower abdomen-into your dan tian-the source of your energy, your chi. Your abdomen holds this glowing ball of energy using this white light to circulate through your body at times you can't concentrate on doing that. It is always there for your body. Always working to your higher good; a source of deep contentment deep within you, always glowing, always healing, always at peace. This is a source of energy you can draw up with just a breath whenever you need to be reminded of the light within you.

Deeply relaxed, body glowing with the brightness of the healing light, know that you are loved. You are special. You are unique in the universe. You are truly beautiful. These are the gifts the light leaves with you. Breathing gently, aware of the peaceful feelings you experienced, you let the light gently fade. You are you. Back to the present. Back to the day-to-day happenings of your life. Now a creature of earth and light, smile and slowly open your eyes. Aware. Alert. Alive.

Chapter Five:
Healing Touch and Other Complementary Therapies

From acupuncture to Zen gardening there are dozens of complementary therapies that offer relaxation, pain relief, and healing outside of traditional Western medicines.

I want to make a special emphasis that my opinion is that they are best used as **complementary** therapies and **not alternative** therapies. Complementary means "mutually making up what is lacking." Alternative means "choice between two or more things." These non-traditional therapies make up what is lacking in traditional Western medicine.

Part II: Heal Yourself

You may find a combination of traditional Western medicines and complementary therapies that benefits your health and well-being. You may choose to abandon or have run out of traditional Western medicine options and only use a complementary therapy as your alternative. Or, you may decide it is all just "voodoo" medicine. Just as I recommended doing your research with your illness, do your research when you consider complementary therapies. The choice is yours to make. There is not one sure therapy that benefits every one every time. Always let your health care practitioners (doctors, nurses, etc.) know when you are using complementary therapies, especially herbal medicines. [Their interactions with chemotherapy or other drugs may not be known or may be known to be harmful.]

My experiences with cancer treatments included a great deal of chemotherapy and continue today with radiation, hormonal drugs (Arimidex) and biophosphonates (Zometa). I choose to **complement** those treatments with meditation, qigong, and healing touch therapy.

Healing touch has worked well for me because it enhances the other energy practice of qigong. "Healing Touch is a bio-field therapy that is an energy-based approach to health and healing. It uses touch to influence the human energy system, specifically the energy field that surrounds the body, and the energy centers that control the energy flow from the energy field to the physical body. These non-invasive techniques that utilize the hands to clear, energize, and balance the human and environmental energy fields thus affecting physical, emotional, mental, and spiritual health and healing. It is based on a heart-centered caring relationship in which the practitioner and client come together energetically to facilitate the client's health and healing. The goal in Healing Touch is to restore harmony and balance in the energy system placing the client in a position to self heal. Healing Touch complements conventional health care and is used in collaboration with other approaches to health and healing."[10]

I know people who have gained tremendous benefits from massage, reflexology, and nutritional/juicing therapies. Because these treatments are rarely covered under traditional health insurance plans, look for low or no cost offerings at the large support networks and community colleges.

Chapter Six: Simplicity

There are as many books on how to simplify your life as there are ways to simplify your life. There are tips to simplify your house, your life-style, your finances, your job, your health, and your personal life. Heck, go back to my chapter on *'Living in the Medical World.'* Building your medical notebook is a "tip" to simplify your medical record keeping. Reduce clutter, reduce the number of credit cards, reduce your magazine subscriptions, and reduce the size of your house. Wait, is simplicity about giving everything up? Of course not. The basic theme of all these books really gets down to enjoying the things that really matter without any clutter.

There I've said it. Neatness is a virtue. Don't sweat the small stuff. How often do we hear the same message over and over again. None of it is new news or even new ways, except maybe the book is cuter or funnier, but not really new.

That is what makes it so profound. Simplicity is simple. It is as basic as saying yes or no to you. It is as basic as knowing the difference between a need and a want. It is as basic as believing that there is no truth in the saying, "A clean desk is a sign of a sick mind." Let your mind be sick! Heck, your body is. (That is, of course, if you have chronic illness.)

You have enough going on that you do need to take those tips and apply them to your life so that you make the daily tasks easier to manage. When you simplify, you have the additional consideration of how your illness limits your physical activities and your finances.

Housework is easier when clutter is reduced. Even when we can afford cleaning help, most of us at least pick up the clutter before the help arrives. When we are fatigued, running errands can be next to impossible. Plan your day to include what has to be done as well as where so that you reduce your "running around" time. Landscaping that was once an enjoyable pastime can

Part II: Heal Yourself

become a burden. Stop planting annuals and find some perennial flowers that you enjoy. If you can afford it, pay to have the grass cut and fertilized. Maybe face the hard question of moving into a community where you no longer have maintenance responsibilities.

Use the less is more when it comes to living with credit cards, e.g. one major credit card can work as well as seven separate department store cards. The same philosophy works with clothing, decorating, banking and investments, eating out and other entertainment options.

The first few steps will be difficult. However, reassess where you were and where you are two months after you've put those simplicity tips into action. I have no doubt that you will think your life is better. When you have chronic illness you are pretty much living on the edge anyway. You do not need all that junk behind you taking up your space and pushing you over. Give yourself a nice wide-open place.

Think of your life as a large mason jar. Inside are some pretty and good-sized stones – the important things in your life. The jar is nice to have around and nice to look at. You can see each stone and appreciate its individual beauty, shape, and color. Then one day, a bunch of pebbles got dumped in the jar. Well, it was

Looking Good Was Never My Problem

okay. You could still see the stones, not as well, but you knew they were there. Pretty soon, though, the jar was filled with sand. The stones were there, but you couldn't tell one lump from the other. You couldn't appreciate the stones. They looked dirty with all that sand. Finally, the jar gets filled with water. Now the sand is muddy. The beautiful stones can't be seen at all. It is just totally gross and you don't like the jar at all.

It is very easy for your life to become that jar when you do not simplify

Chapter Seven:
Purpose and Focus

"Why me?" is one of the first question to haunt cancer patients. Often it takes months for people to grapple with the question before they realize that an answer does not exist.

I never questioned why I got cancer. It is not because I've discovered the non-existent answer to "Why me?" Mostly, I thought "Why not me?" Bad things happen to good people all the time.

"Why me?" became my question a couple of years later. Why didn't I die from IBC? Why did the 18-year-old girl have to die? What about the mother of two young children? Why was I the one to make it five plus years?

Looking Good Was Never My Problem

Let's face it. If I were supposed to solve the Mid East Crisis or find the solution for world hunger, wouldn't I have been on that path a lot earlier? I was an accountant, for Pete's sake; hardly a more noble profession than tax collector. I desperately prayed for a sign – something not too subtle either. I was afraid I was not doing what I was supposed to be doing. I was afraid I was not listening hard enough. What was my purpose?

Our minister provided me with the best answer – live your life so that the light of God shines through whatever you do or say. Three years later, I was still struggling with whether or not I was living my life well enough. I prayed for guidance. The next day, I received an email from our associate pastor asking me to speak to a group of our junior high youth and their parents. The topic was on my personal experiences with prayer.

Focus is a little more difficult. I think it is an inherited trait. I just get so many ideas of things I want to do. My father tends to be the same way. Unfortunately, none of them seem to get finished. I can even get sidetracked on daily tasks. Like almost everything else in life, there have been numerous books, tapes, and videos dealing with focus. What I find most

Part II: Heal Yourself

interesting is that the more you read these "self-help" books, the more you feel like you're watching re-runs on TV. But every once in awhile, you read something you didn't read before. Those are the ideas that stick with you. Those are the ideas you make your own.

My two favorites are the personal mission statement and priority list. I wrote my personal mission statement on September 24, 1998, nearly one year before my diagnosis, and I still like it today.

"To embrace each day with all the passion, wisdom, and joy I've been blessed with. Everyday I will have the courage to share an authentic smile. By being a source of positive energy for others, I will reap the benefits for myself."

Obviously, a personal mission statement doesn't have to be a work of literary genius. Allow your personal mission statement to embrace your purpose and provide a focus for your daily actions. When it works, you will find yourself becoming the person you really want to be.

A priority list can be a lot like a to do list, but better. It is better because it sets the priority, the importance, of what you have to do. A to do list will have "clean the bathrooms" and "take my children to the park." Unless the bathrooms are candidates for a health department violation, a priority list will have only "take my children to the park." Of course, the day will come when "clean the bathrooms" rightly belongs on the priority list.

It is easy to become overwhelmed by an overloaded to do list. I love lists. Oops, now my husband who took great pleasure in leaving me a to do list every day when we were first married, knows the truth. I was just exercising my independence in choosing to ignore his lists. Lists keep you focused. You remember what you need to do. You remember what you need when you run errands so you eliminate the extra trips that tire you. More important, you actually get things done.

My father taught me to carry around a small memo notebook to keep track of what I needed to do that day. Sometimes I would add to that day's list or start on one for tomorrow. At night, I take out my notebook and think about the priorities for the next day – my focus for tomorrow.

Chapter Eight: Five Simple Steps to Heal Yourself

Below are five simple action steps you can take that will enhance your body's ability to heal itself.

Step1: Find the support you need.

An organized support group is your first step. However, if you find that your group focuses too much on the newly diagnosed and those undergoing treatments, you may need to find support from other sources. Living with metastatic cancer is about managing your life differently. You may find your support by working with a local chapter of a national organization or on the Internet, where you have broader exposure to more people also living with metastatic cancer or your illness. Your support may come from family or friends. Remember, you will get what you need when you give of yourself. Find a place to give, and you will find your support.

Step 2: Use your foods and exercise program to build energy.

Food and exercise are the physical things your body needs to function. You have to be able to function to live and have energy. Choose your foods in a way that maximize your energy and health. Basic qigong exercises described in this book will guide your body's natural energy to help you. You may even find that you can participate in classes at your local YMCA or gym.

Step 3: Step out of your "comfort zone" and participate in an alternative healing program.

Healing touch is a safe, non-invasive, complementary therapy that works with the body's natural healing energy. Many doctors, clinics, and cancer centers now embrace the benefits of complementary healing programs when used in conjunction with traditional medical treatments. The idea of managing chronic illness may be as new to your medical team as it is to you. Have the courage to try something new.

Step 4: Simplify your lifestyle

Simplifying your lifestyle is completing a major housecleaning where you do more than clean your house. You clean your life so that you know and live with what you really need. Sure, you have to get rid of the clutter. You have to reduce and streamline your wardrobe, your kitchen pantry, and your decorating. You have to consolidate your finances, travel reward program points, and who knows what else. And in the end, you know you have more even when other people look at you and think you have less. Simplicity must be like one of those carnival mirrors that can take short pudgy people and make them look tall and skinny.

Step 5: Use your spirituality to define your focus and purpose

Spirit, our connection to the great universal good, can guide our lives so that we feel we live with a purpose and with focus. We help Spirit when we have intention. It is easy to let the physical limitations that metastatic disease or chronic illness can put on our bodies influence our spiritual health as well. We can avoid that when we develop our personal mission and focus our lives outside of ourselves. Meditation is one tool we have to stay aligned with Spirit.

To reinforce what you have just read, repeat the following intentions for managing your chronic illness by healing yourself.

*I participate in or develop
my own support network.*

*I make sensible food choices
to enhance my physical energy.*

*I practice qigong exercises and meditate
to enhance my healing energy.*

I am receptive to alternative healing methods.

I simplify my household and activities.

*I am in touch with Spirit
to understand my purpose.*

Part III: Live Your Life

"The warrior's approach is to say "yes" to life; "yea" to it all."
Joseph Campbell

To begin living your life, know that you will have to make changes. Chronic illnesses have a way of limiting your physical mobility and energy levels. Activities with family and friends will change. As long as you are open to that change and embrace it without a great deal of self-pity, you will be able to live!

The key to that acceptance is maintaining a positive attitude. As you will read in the next chapters, positive attitude is the combination of faith and gratitude.

Chapter One:
Lifestyle Adjustments

You do not have to be afraid of cancer. When the disease is diagnosed, treated and goes away, it becomes a "what if," a shadow lurking at the end of the alleyway. When the cancer is diagnosed, treated, but doesn't go away, it becomes a "when." It isn't a shadow but an ever-present fact of life –it has substance and form – at least to the patient.

My metastatic IBC has become a relative who has overstayed her welcome. She's family, so you can't kick her out. Instead, you have to learn to live with her (it).

Friends and family often assume, since I'm not dead, that my cancer is in remission. Remission (as defined by The National Cancer Institute) is a "decrease in or

Part III: Live Your Life

disappearance of signs and symptoms of cancer. In partial remission, some, but not all, signs and symptoms of cancer have disappeared. In complete remission, all signs and symptoms of cancer have disappeared, although cancer still may be in the body." Thankfully the metastasis in the bones is growing slowly, but there is no disappearance.

My cancer is like those little fish that live on whales, except my cancer doesn't provide any benefits. Or, does it? Obviously, from a physical standpoint, no. From a spiritual standpoint, the benefits are numerous.

Facing one's own mortality can be mind boggling, especially when you're young. When you live your life always thinking you'll take care of it "tomorrow," you'll take that trip when you "retire," or "next" Christmas I'll do this or that, you put yourself in, at best, a room with a narrow door and one window. The door barely opens and the window is dirty, grimy, and covered by dingy shades and heavy, dusty draperies. You can't see a thing out of that window. Do you want to know what is outside?

Today. The present. This moment in time. And you can't see any of it. Those nasty cancer cells roaming the bones of my spine, hips, and arm took a detour into my room with the narrow door and one window. They

Looking Good Was Never My Problem

ripped off the heavy draperies, threw away the shades, and Windex-ed the heck out of the glass panes. I now live in a room with a view!

It's not an absolutely perfect view and every once in a while a bird will do his business on the panes. All in all, though, it's a great view. Life with metastatic cancer is better from a room with a view.

There are a few basic changes you may need to make in yourself in order find your view:

- Develop clear intentions of what you want out of life but don't be attached to the outcome.
- Stop judging and start forgiving.
- Live in the moment. Use your senses.
- Laugh.

When our son was a small boy, he had the most unusual luck of finding dimes in the coin returns of pay phones. It never ceased to amaze us how he would find the change left behind in vending machines. He even had the luck of hitting a vending machine with his fist and having a soda or candy bar slide out. It never happened for the rest of us. To this day, I believe it worked for Nathan because he believed it would. He's had some rough patches and disappointments, but he still says, "See, Mom, I told you I'd turn out

Part III: Live Your Life

okay." And, he has. He has always believed he will be successful and happy. His secret: intend the positive – intending to be a success is different from intending not to be a failure.

Live with a positive intention. Intend to be healthy and happy. Intend to interact with family and friends. Intend to follow your exercise and meditation program. Believe that you are capable of doing all that you intend. But don't get attached to the outcome. I'd be lying if I didn't admit that I intend all these positive things because I want to live longer and live better. The satisfaction isn't in the outcome. Your satisfaction must come from the doing.

This leads us to living in the moment. To live in the moment, you have first to throw away that giant trash bag you carry around filled with the garbage of the past. What if we all really had to carry our pasts with us in large black trash bags? What would a crowded city street look like, your office building, the shopping mall? Imagine cheering your child at soccer or leading their scout troop or even snuggling on the sofa with your loved one with a giant black trash bag or two tied around you. Seems ridiculous, right? So why do we do it?

Two reasons – we don't forgive and we judge.

Let's make it perfectly clear – forgiving is not the same as forgetting. We'll go back to the dictionary.

To forgive means to give up resentment against.

To forget means to be unable to remember.

Rarely do we lose memory of things that happen. Actually, at least my experience is that I remember best either the wrong or hateful things I've done or had done to me better than I remember the good things. I think trying to forget would be a waste of energy because the success rate would be too low.

But trying to forgive – now that would be a glorious accomplishment. To forgive truly means that you can say the following:

> "I no longer resent you for either who you are or what you did."

> "I know that I am not responsible for your actions or feelings, only how I feel or act about them."

When you are able to forgive, you have the personal freedom to be kind to yourself. Resentment can fill up those black trash bags very quickly. You just don't need it. Resentment and anger can eat away at you as badly as any cancer can.

If forgiveness is so great, wouldn't forgetting be great too? No, forgetting will not always allow you to

Part III: Live Your Life

accept responsibility for your own actions and feelings, i.e. how you feel about someone else's actions. You don't want to forget, for example, a situation that was physically or emotional neglectful or abusive. In the same way that you learn not to touch a hot stove (i.e. a hot stove can burn and burns can hurt), your remembering protects you. It warns you to stay away from those situations. You are responsible for your feelings and actions so you need to have a frame of reference in which to accept that responsibility.

Once you learn to forgive, it is quite natural to stop judging. By judging, I mean evaluating why someone doesn't measure up to what I think they should be. Why aren't my friends more supportive? Why don't my spouse/parents/children love me more?

I'll use my own family to make two illustrations on how judgments could have ruined our relationships.

[1] When I was in the hospital for four weeks getting HDC/SCT, my father never came to see me. Did this mean he didn't love me? Did this mean he didn't care that I was sick? I could have made the judgment that his behavior indicated that he didn't care, but I didn't. Here was a man in his mid-seventies, married for over fifty years.

He gave his wife (my mother) up for four weeks so she could stay with me. That is an amazing sacrifice that only a man with a great deal of love for both his child and her mother could make.

[2] Twenty-three years into my marriage and I finally understood (also while in that hospital on our wedding anniversary) what love is all about. Why hadn't I understood before? Because I was judging my husband's actions against my expectations and predetermined notions of what love was supposed to be. When I stopped comparing what he was able to give me against what I thought love was supposed to be, I realized I had love. I had all the love he had to give. I had it all. How much more could I expect?

Suddenly, I was seeing all kinds of relationships in a new light. I had really good friends that had a hard time accepting my illness. They kept their distance. Other people, who I would have thought of as more casual acquaintances, really stepped up and did a lot to help. Was one a better friend than the other? This isn't a judgment I am willing to make. Friends, like family,

Part III: Live Your Life

give you what they can. Don't judge their actions to determine their value as friends. Embrace whatever gifts people have to give you. Don't be critical.

If you find the gifts (love/support) from family/friends/caregivers is not enough, then you must look inside yourself to identify what it is you need. You can't expect other people to know what it is. You can't be disappointed that you don't have it, if you haven't asked for it. Remember, it is your responsibility to take care of your actions and feelings. That may mean taking action to find what you need from other people. Judging and criticizing the people you know will not enable them to give you something they just don't have to begin with.

You will start to see a more colorful, unique world around you when you no longer judge. What is really neat is that you see yourself better too. It is a win-win situation or a buy one / get one free sale. It is often said that the more you give to life, the more you will get in return. It is also true that the way you look at the world around you changes how you see yourself and how the world sees you. These are all good changes.

Once you've made these changes, you'll be able to laugh at yourself too. Laughter, whether at a comedy club or at your own inadequacies and mistakes, is truly the best medicine. I love to laugh. I always have. Some people are given gifts of musical, athletic, or artistic talents. I laugh.

Watch the movie *Roger Rabbit*. There is a scene in which the cartoon, Roger Rabbit, is handcuffed to the live actor private investigator, Eddie Valiant. They go through several scenes where their being handcuffed together gets them into some tight spots, all of which are handled with a lot of comedy. It isn't until the very end, when Eddie is finally able to saw the handcuffs off, that Roger Rabbit very calmly pulls his hand out of the cuff. Eddie is stunned. "You mean you could have pulled your hand out earlier?" "No," Roger Rabbit replied, "only when it was funny.". Now, that is the way to live life. I just love that scene.

Of course, I will probably end up like the weasels in *Roger Rabbit* and die laughing. I can think of worse ways to go.

A better way, though, would be dancing - another great thing to enjoy in life. My husband and I would rate about a two on a scale of one-to-ten, and that is if we really stretch it. However, in terms of enjoyment, we are off the scale. Those are the changes you can make; of course, you don't have to have metastatic cancer or a chronic illness to make them. However, if you do have cancer, then make the changes so you can live!

Your Career

I changed employers after my initial treatment. My new employer was not aware of my diagnosis. When the metastasis was discovered, I had to start all over again with how much information to share and whom to share it with. This is often difficult, especially since so many people still see cancer as a death sentence. You'll get the folks who want to "mother" you, the ones who avoid you, and the ones who resent the fact that you may leave early or come in late. When I reduced my work hours by 50%, the people who did not know the reason considered me to be something of a "princess" who just didn't want to work that hard. To deal with this, try to let go of your reputation.

As Dr. Wayne Dyer advises in <u>The Power of Intention</u>, "Your reputation is not located in you. It resides in the minds of others. Therefore, you have no control over it at all. Connecting to intention means listening to your heart and conducting yourself based on what your inner voice tells you is your purpose here. If you're overly concerned with how you're going to be perceived by everyone, then you've disconnected yourself from intention and allowed the opinions of others to guide you. This is your ego at work. Do what you do because your inner voice so directs you."

Your Friends

Accept the fact that, no matter how weird or stupid some people seem, they truly think their words and actions are well intentioned.

For example, after returning to classes after the summer break, one of my daughter's classmates asked her, "Is your mom dead yet?"

Then there's the comment and reply that prompted the title of this book.

"Oh, you look so good."

"Looking good was never my problem."

(especially effective using a Mae West accent.)

A friend who suffers from both asthma and fibromalygia gave me this one:

When questioned about her need for a handicap-parking sticker, a co-worker stated, "You don't look handicapped."

My friend replied, "You don't look stupid either."

Even when you truly accept, follow, and project the "suck it up and deal with it" attitude to whatever the next course of treatment is, most of your friends still

Part III: Live Your Life

won't get it. When my daughter told her friends I was going in for my fourth round of radiation treatments, they didn't understand why she wasn't crying and carrying on. In our house, it is just another two weeks of "spot welding." It doesn't diminish the seriousness of it, but the coping mechanisms you and your family use, may not be understood by your casual friends.

When your illness results in mobility concerns and fatigue, your pattern of social interaction may also change. Crowded restaurants and late dinners just don't work. Are you part of a group of friends that regularly go out for dinner at 7 pm then to the nine o'clock movie? Waiting 30 minutes for a table in the back of a crowded restaurant may not work well if you have difficulty standing or walking. You may be too tired to enjoy your meal. You may fall asleep during the movie. Ask your friends if they can change the schedule. Take advantage of matinees and early-bird specials. Your social group may have to change if your friends are not willing to change with you.

Chapter Two:
Love, Sex, and Intimacy

If you were hoping to get *a true confessions* or *kiss-and-tell story*, I'm sorry to disappoint you. However, any way you look at it, cancer and other degenerative diseases will impact your personal relationships.

For every case where a husband stood by his wife, for example, having an allergic reaction to an antibiotic – naked, missing one breast, tubes and IVs coming out of her, covered with the remnants of hours of vomiting and diarrhea, nearly falling over from rapidly dropping blood pressure – and says "Lean on me" and holds her in the warm shower and helps her get into a clean hospital gown, when he could have just called a nurse into help, there are the husbands who won't even take their wife to the hospital for her mastectomy or, worse,

Part III: Live Your Life

leave the family the day after Christmas because he just can't handle it anymore.

I can't imagine anything more painful than finding out the relationship you believed to be "for better or worse" is not grounded in love. Equally sad is the relationship that ends for lack of a "boob." Surely there's a reason "boob" also means "a stupid fellow". Fortunately, I did not have to deal with either.

All that aside, even in the best of relationships, sex can become complicated, or, at the very least, require some changes. For example, during chemotherapy, I got this warning "It is possible that traces of chemotherapy are also present in vaginal fluid and semen. A condom should be worn during sexual intercourse within 72 hours after you or your sexual partner receive chemotherapy." Using condoms had not been part of our relationship since I'd had a tubal ligation nearly 18 years earlier.

Chemotherapies can throw women into early menopause, lessening sexual desire and making sex uncomfortable. It is important to accept this as a natural aging process that just happened earlier than you expected. Talk to your doctor about what you can do.

Many patients take anti-depressants. Let's be honest, even with the best of attitudes, dealing with pain or a weakening body isn't easy. Unfortunately, one of the side effects may be lessened sexual desire. Again, if you notice this change, talk to your doctor.

Sex is between you and your partner. What you develop as a mutually satisfying relationship is between you (and what you choose to share with your health professional). What works for you, may not be the same as what works for your best girlfriend or me but, always communicate your needs and be receptive to communication from your husband or partner about his or her needs too.

Intimacy is not to be mistaken with sex. Because of pain or difficulty sleeping, couples may choose to sleep in separate beds or bedrooms. This isn't a lack of love or even a lack of desire, but a respect for each other's needs. What it can lead to, though, is a loss of intimacy. Human beings need intimacy, touch, and comfort. Do not give up those kisses good-by or good night, the genuine glad-to-see-you hugs after work, and some snuggle time on the sofa watching old movies. Quiet moments of intimacy nurture the loving foundation of a relationship. They provide opportunities for communication, to share fears and dreams.

Don't waste opportunities to say "I love you" or give a friend a hug.

Chapter Three:
Attitude Is Everything

"Every thought you have has an energy that will either strengthen or weaken you."[11]

I cannot tell you how many people have commented on my positive attitude. A positive attitude is nothing more than knowing that you are loved.

Staying connected to God (Spirit) is key to maintaining a positive attitude. Stress, illness, disappointing test results, fear, family pressures, and financial strains can all manifest themselves to pull you down. One day of self-pity can turn into two, then three, then a week, and before you know it, the positive attitude is lost.

The simplest way to stay connected is never to lose sight of what you have to be thankful for. In her book,

Part III: Live Your Life

<u>Simple Abundance</u>, Sarah Ban Breathnach recommends keeping a Gratitude Journal. The type of book you use isn't important, but it is nice to find one that helps put you into a pleasant frame of mind. I used a simple spiral notepad with a motivational quote on the cover: "Some people dream of success… while others wake up and work hard at it." I don't think that had anything to do with gratitude. More likely, the notepad was in the clearance rack at a local store. However, it served its purpose.

For me, it is important to view the end of each day as a new beginning. To stay connected, I end the day with my focus on at least one thing that I have to be thankful for. I refuse to let my focus be on any negative thoughts. Even if all I feel I can be thankful for is a bed to sleep in, I focus on that.

Keep that focus on thank **you** – not thank **me**. Know that there is a higher being in charge, providing, taking care of, loving, reminding you that you are not dealing with this illness alone.

<u>Faith</u>

Religion has long been man's answer to what he didn't understand. Ancient Greek and Roman gods provided answers for natural phenomena we now scientifically understand.

With all of our scientific advances and discoveries, death remains a mystery. Today we still turn to religion for our answers to what we do not understand.

Whether you believe in God, the Source, or Spirit it is defined, at www.freedictinary.com, to mean the vital principle or animating force within living beings, incorporeal consciousness, the soul, or the part of a human associated with the mind, will, and feelings

I choose to believe in God and Jesus – the Christian faith. I do not intend for this to be a conversion document, but an explanation of where Christianity and faith fit into living with my metastatic disease. If you have a belief that gives you comfort, answers, strength, and peace that is wonderful. If you are searching for all of that, please read on.

God loves me. God loves you. As a child, I learned the song "Jesus Loves Me."

> Jesus loves me, this I know
> For the Bible tells me so.
> Little ones to him belong,
> They are weak but He is strong.

Part III: Live Your Life

    Yes, Jesus loves me.

    Yes, Jesus loves me.

    Yes, Jesus loves me.

    The Bible tells me so.

It is amazing how much comfort this children's song brought an adult while at the brink of death.

You are God's creation, and in His eyes you are blessed. Through Jesus, you are forgiven all your sins. By His grace, you are accepted. Even when the rest of the world is too busy, God is there for you. We all need to be loved. No matter how much you may be rejected by family and friends, God will never reject you. What a wonderful piece of knowledge – you are loved, accepted and forgiven just the way you are.

Through the community of faith, we can share God's love through prayer. I have been on prayer lists at churches of various denominations all over the country. Through these prayers, I've felt myself surrounded by what I envisioned to be a "love bubble". I was inside the bubble, protected by all the prayers. Don't be afraid to share God's love through prayers for others. As you struggle with your deteriorating health and physical limitations, it helps to gain comfort from the "love bubble."

Looking Good Was Never My Problem

Jesus' messages and the words of his apostles give me hope and encouragement. A friend of mine once shared that she didn't want to die. I asked her if it was because she was afraid of death. It is good not to want to die. God did not provide us with so many wonderful things and expect us to want to die. However, you will die. You will not choose how or when, but you will die. You don't have to be afraid of death. God has prepared a place for you.

Blessed be the God and Father of our Lord Jesus Christ! By his mercy he has given us a new birth into a long hope through the resurrection of Jesus Christ from the dead, and into an inheritance that is imperishable, undefiled, and unfading, kept in heaven for you, who are being protected by the power of God through faith for a salvation ready to be revealed in the last time. In this you rejoice, even if now for a little while you have had to suffer various trials, so that the genuineness of your faith – being more precious than gold that, though perishable, is tested by fire – may be found to result in praise and glory and honor when Jesus Christ is revealed. Although you have not seen him, you love him; and even

Part III: Live Your Life

though you do not see him now, you believe in him and rejoice with an indescribable and glorious joy, for you are receiving the outcome of your faith, the salvation of your souls.
1st Peter, verses 3–9,

Holy Bible, New Revised Standard Version

We have so many gifts on earth; I cannot imagine there would be less in heaven.

Gratitude

Sarah Ban Breathnach writes in her book, Simple Abundance,

"What is missing from many of our days is a true sense that we are enjoying the lives we are living. It is difficult to experience moments of happiness if we are not aware of what it is we genuinely love. We must learn to savor small, authentic moments that bring us contentment. Experiment with a new cookie recipe. Take the time to slowly arrange a bouquet of flowers in order to appreciate their colors, fragrance, and beauty. Sip a cup of tea on the front stoop in the sunshine. Pause for five minutes to pet a purring cat. Simple pleasures waiting to be enjoyed. Simple pleasures often overlooked."

Looking Good Was Never My Problem

While I write at my computer, moose surround me. Fifty stuffed moose of various sizes, colors, and expressions line the shelves and bookcases, tables and television top of my room. Not as frou-frou as a bouquet of flowers, but I even have a chocolate scented one. Moose make me laugh. I've never even seen a real moose, but these stuffed ones with their big faces and gangly legs and knobby knees are funny. Moose are undoubtedly the most often overlooked simple pleasure in the universe.

We spend far too much energy whining and moaning about what we don't have that we lose sight of what we do have. How often, when asked if they were told they only had six months to live, people choose to spend that time in the simple, daily tasks and joys of life. Playing board games, going for long walks, watching the sunset, spending time with family and friends. There are dozens of simple pleasures waiting to be enjoyed.

Faith + Gratitude = Positive Attitude

When you are able to combine your faith with gratitude you will have the attitude you need to live your life with a chronic illness. God provides us every blessing in abundance. God provides us with love.

Part III: Live Your Life

When we come to realize that we have all that we need – all the love, all the beauty, all the grace -- we no longer see life as a vacuum waiting to be filled. Instead, life becomes an overflowing garden of tomatoes, zucchini, and cucumbers that we are more than willing to leave on the counter for anyone to take. We feel no need to hold back. We are free to give and to love because we know that we will always have an abundance of love and whatever else we need.

Our chronic illness no longer scares us because it is no longer the focus of our life. Our attitude transcends the fear and replaces it with love. When we begin and end our day in a state of gratitude and love, we no longer judge others or ourselves. We are free.

In my gratitude journal I am grateful for my family, chocolate chip cookies, the sunshine, my friends, and smiley faces. I am grateful for my moose, the geese that come to live in the field behind our house, the monarch butterfly at our butterfly bush, hearing my daughter play the piano, and my son's telephone calls.

I am grateful that I am loved just the way I am.

Repeat that sentence over and over again until you too can say it with tears in your eyes and a smile on your face. Thank you, God, I am so very, very lucky.

Chapter Four:
Five Simple Steps to Managing Life with Cancer

Below are five simple steps to help manage the day-to-day challenges of life with cancer.

Step 1: Accept the changes that happen to and in you.

Change is scary. Change management is an entire business discipline. Metastatic cancer can change you into an angry, bitter person unable to find a speck of joy in your life. Metastatic cancer can also open your eyes and your heart to a world so spectacular, so colorful, and so creative that you, too, feel moved to write a poem about something as simple as the colors you see while walking the dog.

*Part III: *Live Your Life*

Primary Colors

The light blue sky surrounded the
tiny yellow butterfly as it landed
on the deep yellow dandelion –
A solitary stem protruding in the
middle of the freshly mown field
of green weeds.
A pair of black crows nose-dived into
the swaying stalks of green corn in
the field nearby.
A mottled brown bunny flashed his
fluffy white cottontail and disappeared
after the black crows.
All while my dog sniffed at the red fire hydrant
across the dirty white sidewalk
that runs alongside the field
of green weeds.

Step 2: Understand that changes will happen in your relationships.

Just as you'll experience changes within yourself, you'll experience changes in your personal and professional relationships. Changes may draw people closer to you or push people away. Remember that you cannot make someone feel or act a certain way. You have to accept these changes and move on.

Step 3: Truly believe that you are loved.

Even if there is no one else, God loves you. If you don't want to believe in God, then the universe loves you. Every unique combination of cells in your body is loved. Your soul is part of the collective universe. You belong. You are loved.

Step 4: Stay in focus with a positive attitude and lots of gratitude.

A positive attitude is a choice. It is a choice you make by staying in focus with your purpose. It is a choice you make by acknowledging all the blessings in your life every day. Don Miguel Ruiz in his book, The Four Agreements, writes:

"But there is really no reason to suffer. The only reason you suffer is because you choose to suffer. If you look at your life you will find many excuses to suffer, but a good reason to suffer you will not find. The same is true for happiness. The only reason you are happy is because you choose to be happy. Happiness is a choice, and so is suffering.

Maybe we cannot escape from the destiny of the human, but we have a choice: to suffer our destiny or to enjoy our destiny. To suffer, or to love and be happy."

Step 5: If you've lost it, find your faith. If you have it, take strength from it.

I am very happy with my Christian faith. If your faith is in another religion, that is great too. If you don't have a religious or traditional faith, I hope that you can find, at the least, an acceptance of Spirit, a greater good, or something stronger than you. When the day is done and you've faced your challenges and changes, when you've recognized all the blessings in your life, you can close your eyes and not be alone in the darkness. Instead of darkness, you see a warm light reaching toward you, embracing you, and quietly saying, "You are loved."

To reinforce what you have just read, repeat the following intentions for living your life.

I will experience changes in the way I look at life.
I choose to accept those changes
with a positive attitude.

I will experience changes in my relationships with family and friends. I choose to accept those changes with a positive attitude.

I say "thank you" every day for even the smallest blessings in my life.

When I combine my faith with gratitude, I live with a positive attitude.

I am loved.

Epilogue

I first saw the term "warrior" applied to cancer patients on the website for inflammatory breast cancer support. Even though it is five years since diagnosis, I do not think of myself as a survivor. My cancer isn't gone. I am still fighting it. I am still a warrior.

"How are we to become a warrior? ~~There are certain characteristics of the warrior that are nearly the same around the world.~~ The warrior has awareness. The warrior has control. To refrain is to hold the emotions and to express them in the right moment, not before, not later. That is why warriors are impeccable. They have complete control over their own emotions and therefore over their own behavior." *(Ruiz)*

Warrior Women

"You join an army of wounded women, who wear pretty clothes that conceal the scars and the pain and who summon brave smiles to camouflage anxiety. We each share a touching, intimate memory of a day that changed our lives forever.

Each precious moment on this earth is a gift. We will not leave this gift unopened. We will not leave one smile undone. We will not leave one hug forgotten. We will not miss one opportunity to make a difference.

We are Women Warriors. Our casualties are high. The women who have gone before us have lost a battle with breast cancer, but they haven't lost the war.

We have breast cancer. We are alive."

Author Unknown, excerpt from IBC Warrior's Site, www.ibcsupport.org

"I am not dying from cancer; I am living with it.

Ellen Stahl

Acknowledgements

I would like to acknowledge Lorie Allen, my sister and friend, who contributed so much to the sections on exercise, meditation, and healing touch. I cannot thank her enough for finding her healing gift because she wanted to help her "baby sister."

To my support team, my husband, Wayne, my children, Nathan and Sarah, and my parents, Robert and Beverly Jenner, thank you so much for the encouragement. You are the best caregivers and have always been there when I needed you throughout my journey.

Special thanks are also extended to Donna, Melody and Beth for acting as readers and editors.

For my beloved dog, Molly, our Golden Retriever, who taught me so much about life – like stretching before you get up, eating what is put in front of you and being thankful for it, enjoying long walks, loving and accepting without judgment, and wanting nothing more in life than to snuggle up with the people you love. When we had to put Molly to sleep while I was writing this book, she taught me that there can and should be dignity and laughter in death as there is in life.

References and Resources

References

[1] National Institutes of Health, National Cancer Institute. "What You Need To Know About Breast Cancer." NIH Publication No. 98-1556, Revised August 1998. Printed September 1998.

[2] Source: http://www.uslegalforms.com/living-will-forms.htm

[3] Source: http://www.uslegalforms.com/living-will-forms.htm

[4] Source: http://www.alcoholicsvictorious.org/supp-faq.html#what

[5] Source: WebMD and AOL Health – Cancer-Related Fatigue

[6] Cohen, Kenneth S. The Way of Qigong. New York: Ballantine Books, 1997

[7] *News-Gazette*, Champaign, Illinois, July 9, 2004

[8] Dyer, Wayne W. The Power of Intention. Hay House, Inc., 2004

[9] Chopra D., and David Simon. Grow Younger, Live Longer. New York: Harmony Books, 2001.

[10] Source: www.healingtouch.net

[11] Dyer: The Power of Intention.

Resources

American Cancer Society. http://www.cancer.org/

Ban Breathnach, Sarah. *Simple Abundance*. New York: Warner Books, 1995.

Chopra D., and David Simon. *Grow Younger, Live Longer*. New York

Harmony Books, 2001.

Cohen, Kenneth S. *The Way of Qigong*. New York: Ballantine Books, 1997.

Dyer, Wayne W. *The Power of Intention: Learning to Co-Create Your World Your Way*. Carlsbad, California: Hay House, 2004.

Dyer, Wayne W. *10 Secrets for Success and Inner Peace*. Carlsbad, California: Hay House, 2004.

HH Dalai Lama and Howard C. Cutler, M.D. *The Art of Happiness*. New York: Riverhead Books. 1998.

HH Dalai Lama and Renuka Singh, ed. *Live in a Better Way*. New York: Penguin Books. 1999.

Johnson, Spencer. *The Precious Present*. New York: Doubleday. 1984

Lu, Nan. *A Natural Guide to Weight Loss That Lasts*. New York: Harper Collins Publishers. 2000

Lu, Nan. *A Woman's Guide to Healing from Breast Cancer*. New York: Avon Books. 1999.

Ruiz, Don Miguel. *The Four Agreements*. San Rafael, California: Amber-Allen Publishing, 1997.

Siegel, Bernie S. *Love, Medicine and Miracles : Lessons Learned about Self-Healing from a Surgeon's Experience with Exceptional Patients*. New York: Harper Collins Publishers, 1986.

Siegel, Bernie S. *Meditations for Enhancing Your Immune System: Strengthen Your Body's Ability to Heal*. Audio cassette or CD.

Susan G. Komen Breast Cancer Foundation. http://www.komen.org

St. James, Elaine. *Simplify Your Life*. New York: Hyperion, 1994.

Warren, Rick. *The Purpose Driven Life*. Grand Rapids: Zondervan, 2002.

About the Authors

Ellen Stahl has been living with metastatic breast cancer for over five years. With an original prognosis of less than two years to live, she has amazed family, friends, and medical professionals with her positive attitude. She's seen her daughter graduate college; her son graduate college and get married; and traveled with her husband. Ellen's own experiences and those of close friends coping with multiple sclerosis, fibromyalgia, back injury, and cancer inspired her to share her own journey and life lessons in this book

Lorie Allen, Ellen's sister, is a healing touch practitioner apprentice. Lorie's desire to help Ellen and others has resulted in an amazing discovery of her healing gift. She also teaches relaxation, meditation, and stress management techniques.

Printed in the United States
81272LV00001B/187-192